Auditing
Physician Services:

Verifying Accuracy in Physician Services and E/M Coding to Protect Medical Practices

— SECOND EDITION —

BETSY NICOLETTI, MS, CPC

Founder, Codapedia.com

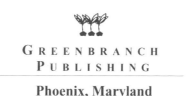

GREENBRANCH
PUBLISHING

Phoenix, Maryland

Copyright © 2015 by Greenbranch Publishing, LLC
ISBN 978-0-9907241-5-5
eISBN 978-0-9907241-6-2

Published by Greenbranch Publishing, LLC
PO Box 208
Phoenix, MD 21131
Phone: (800) 933-3711
Fax: (410) 329-1510
Email: info@greenbranch.com
Websites: www.greenbranch.com, www.soundpractice.net, www.codapedia.com

Greenbranch Publishing books are available at special quantity discounts to use as premiums and sales promotions, or for use in corporate training programs. For more information, please write to the Director of Special Sales, Greenbranch Publishing, PO Box 208, Phoenix, MD 21131 or (800) 933-3711 or info@ greenbranch.com.

This publication is designed to provide general medical practice management information and is sold with the understanding that neither the author nor the publisher is engaged in rendering legal, accounting, ethical, or clinical advice. While all information in this document is believed to be correct at the time of writing, no warranty, express or implied, is made as to its accuracy as information may change over time. If legal or other expert advice is required, the services of a competent professional person should be sought.

CPT® is a registered trademark of the American Medical Association

PUBLISHER
Nancy Collins

EDITORIAL ASSISTANT
Jennifer Weiss

BOOK DESIGNER
Laura Carter
Carter Publishing Studio

COPYEDITOR
Robert A. Saigh

INDEXER
Robert A. Saigh

Table of Contents

This book is dedicated to my fellow auditors.
They say stress doesn't cause gray hair, but we know better.

About the Author

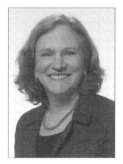

Betsy Nicoletti, MS, CPC, is the co-founder of Codapedia, a Web site devoted to physician coding and reimbursement (www.codapedia.com). She has extensive auditing experience in physician services, ensuring that code selection accurately reflects the services performed.

Joking that she is in the "protection" business, Betsy explains that her mission is to simplify complex coding and reimbursement rules for medical practices, thereby "protecting" physician practices. She is the author of *The Field Guide to Physician Coding*, now in its third edition, and *Everyday Medical Coding*, as well as a regular journal contributor. Betsy also speaks to groups on the national scene. When speaking to clinicians, she engages them with an in-depth knowledge of their professional lives. When speaking to fellow auditors, she guides them through the nuances of finding black and white answers in a morass of gray guidelines.

Betsy, who began her consulting business in 1999, has a master's degree in Organization and Management from Antioch New England and is a Certified Professional Coder. She is a member of the Medical Group Management Association and the National Speakers Association. She lives in New England with her dog. Betsy can be reached at www.betsynicoletti.com. Her books are available at www.greenbranch.com and Amazon.com. You can read her blog at www.nicolettinotes.com.

**Download Audit Worksheets at http://auditing2.greenbranch.com
Access code printed on page 195 of this book**

Medical Practice Compliance and the OIG Workplan

At a recent seminar, a general surgeon asked how she could avoid compliance risk when billing Medicare. Before I could answer, the doctor next to her responded, "Don't bill Medicare." Funny and true, but medical practices need a less draconian method of assessing and minimizing risk. The purpose of this book is just that: to give medical practices strategies and tools to reduce the compliance risk related to coding and reimbursement rules. Medical practices cannot avoid risk but can reduce risk by understanding complex coding and reimbursement rules and auditing their documentation for services.

Risk is not limited to Medicare, of course. All government and private payers constantly monitor medical claims for errors, fraud, and abuse. All have instituted claims editing programs to prevent improper payments before the claim is paid, and many are substituting pre-payment audits for "pay and chase." All have implemented software that assesses claim patterns that are different from the norm for other physicians of the same specialty. This can include using CPT® codes at an unusual frequency or pattern, use of modifiers, or sheer volume of services submitted.

How can medical practices protect themselves in an era of increased government and payer compliance scrutiny? In three ways: by focusing on high-risk activities, by performing valid audits, and by conducting reliable, reproducible audit results. A practice that is successful in these three ways can significantly reduce its compliance risk.

Focusing on high-risk activities for audit is the first step after developing a compliance plan. Decide what to audit. It is not necessary to audit the same type of services each year, or to audit the same services for each provider. Rather, a group can assess its own risk areas and select services to audit based on the volume of services provided in any one category and on a review of areas payers or the government have determined to have high risk. It is easy for a group to identify both of these types of service.

Start with volume. Given a choice in auditing a service that is performed twice a week and one performed 100 times a week, select the service with the higher volume. Select services with high relative value units, whether performed frequently or infrequently. Review utilization of Evaluation and Management (E/M) services and use of modifiers. Next, review the current Office of Inspector General (OIG) targets and Recovery Audit Contractor (RAC) areas of interest. Comparing the list of high-frequency services and OIG and RAC targets will provide more than enough areas to audit in a year. Select services that are reported with modifiers that affect payment.

For each area identified, review the coding and reimbursement rules before starting to audit. Some of these common areas are included in this book. If your list includes topics in the book, you are in luck. Review the rules in the chapter and use the audit sheet. In every audit, we strive for both reliability and validity. Reliability means the results are consistent, that the same results would be obtained time after time. That is, if you measured a variable on Monday and used the same test to measure the variable on Wednesday, you would have the same results. Validity is a test of whether you are measuring what you say you are measuring. I strongly urge practices to use an audit tool for all audits, because it increases both validity and reliability. Use the educational resources and audit tools in this book as short cuts. The rules are clearly described and condensed into easy-to-use audit sheets. This will help you focus your scarce compliance resources in areas that are the most relevant for many practices and of high risk from an OIG point of view.

There is no substitute for source documentation. When in doubt, check the Centers for Medicare & Medicaid Services (CMS) website or your Medicare administrative contractor's website. The road to compliance is paved with source citations. And CPT, developed by the American Medical Association, is the source for coding rules.

The OIG is a federally mandated institution created to protect the integrity of the programs of the Department of Health and Human Services (HHS), the welfare of the people HHS serves, and our tax dollars:

> The mission of the Office of Inspector General, as mandated by Public Law 95–452 (as amended), is to protect the integrity of Department of Health and Human Services (HHS) programs, as well as the health and welfare of the beneficiaries of those programs. The OIG has a responsibility to report both to the Secretary and to the Congress program and management problems and recommendations to correct them. The OIG's duties are carried out through a nationwide network of audits, investigations, inspections and other mission-related functions performed by OIG components.

According to the statement of Organization, Function and Delegations of Authority published in the July 2, 2004 *Federal Register*, the activities of the OIG in carrying out this mission are:

- Conducting and supervising audits, investigations, and inspections;
- Identifying systemic weaknesses that create the opportunity for fraud and abuse;
- Leading and coordinating activities to prevent and detect fraud;
- Detecting wrongdoers and abuses; and
- Keeping the Secretary of HHS and the Congress informed of problems.

The OIG Work Plan is published most Octobers. Many OIG departments coordinate their efforts to develop the annual Work Plan, including the Office of Audit Services, the Office of Management and Policy, the Office of Investigations, and the Office of Counsel to the Inspector General. The Work Plan is published in the Publications section of the OIG website, along with the plans from previous years.

The Work Plan is divided into about 20 sections covering Medicare and Medicaid, hospitals, nursing homes, home health, drug pricing, and physician services. This book covers only the Medicare Physicians and Other Health Professionals section. In 2010, the physician section was relabeled as Other Part A and Part B Providers Payments, and that is where a medical practice should look to identify areas the OIG believes are high risk. The OIG Work Plan lists projects started the year before and new starts, along with an expected release date for the report. Some topics appear and then are repeated years later.

The OIG is not only monitoring how accurately medical suppliers and practices are submitting claims; it also is monitoring how effective the Medicare administrative contractors (MACs) are at their administrative functions. The 2015 Work Plan includes new reviews and reviews started in the previous year. 2015 continues the trend of reviewing high-cost diagnostic tests, including diagnostic radiology, imaging serivces and independent lab services.

When the OIG reports are issued, the reports include specific recommendations to Medicare to improve the accuracy of claims payment. Sleep testing is on the list. Both chiropractic and PT services are under scrutiny. And, a perennial favorite, place of service errors. A report released in May 2012 regarding coding trends of E/M services advised CMS to increase education and audits of these services, particularly for 1700 physicians identified as billing the two highest levels of codes in each category more than 95% of the time.

The topics from the 2015 Work Plan are listed below. The OIG, of course, is only one government agency reviewing coding. In 2011, the Justice Department reported recovering a "record-breaking" $4.1 billion in healthcare fraud, estimating that it returns $7.20 for every dollar spent. The OIG estimates it recovers $17.60 for every dollar it spends on enforcement. Not a bad return on investment.

The discussion would not be complete, however, without mentioning the Recovery Audit Contractor (RAC) Initiative. Through this program, CMS hired four private companies to recover monies incorrectly paid to healthcare providers. Using proprietary analytic software, the RACs analyze paid claims data and initiate automated and complex reviews using CMS policies. The RACs are required to post their targets prior to starting a review. The RACs are paid a percentage of the monies they return to the US Trust Fund. In September 2012, one RAC, Connolly Inc., which has the contract for the southeastern states, noted that it would audit three physicians for consistent use of 99215. This is the RACs' first foray into E/M coding, and it raised alarm bells, coming after the E/M coding trends report in May, and along with press reports that using an electronic health record increased the level of E/M services provided in Emergency Departments.

It isn't possible to avoid risk, but it is possible to manage it.

OIG WORK PLAN 2015

Other Providers—Billing and Payments

Acronyms and Abbreviations for Selected Terms Used in This Section:

ASC—ambulatory surgical center
CERT—Comprehensive Error Rate Testing (program)
E/M—evaluation and management (services)
ESRD—end stage renal disease
HOPD—hospital outpatient department
PHP—partial hospitalization program
POD—physician-owned distributor
PPS—prospective payment system
RHC—rural health clinic

Ambulance services—Questionable billing, medical necessity, and level of transport

We will examine Medicare claims data to assess the extent of questionable billing for ambulance services, such as transports that potentially never occurred or potentially were medically unnecessary transports to dialysis facilities. We will also determine whether Medicare payments for ambulance services were made in accordance with Medicare requirements. Prior OIG work found that Medicare made inappropriate payments for advanced life support emergency transports. Medicare pays for emergency and nonemergency ambulance services when a beneficiary's medical condition at the time of transport is such that other means of transportation are contraindicated (i.e., would endanger the beneficiary). (Social Security Act, § 1861(s)(7).) Medicare pays for different levels of ambulance service, including Basic Life Support and Advanced Life Support as well as specialty care transport. (42 CFR § 410.40(b).) (OEI; 09-12-00351; 09-12-00353; expected issue date: FY 2015; and OAS; W-00-11-35574; W-00-12-35574; W-00-13-35574; W-00-14-35574; various
reviews; expected issue date: FY 2015)

Ambulance services—Portfolio report on Medicare Part B payments

We will analyze and synthesize OIG evaluations, audits, investigations, and compliance guidance related to ground ambulance transport services paid by Medicare Part B to identify vulnerabilities, inefficiencies, and fraud trends and offer recommendations to improve detected vulnerabilities and minimize inappropriate payments for ambulance services. Prior OIG work identified fraud schemes and trends indicating overuse and medically unnecessary payments. The planned portfolio will offer recommendations to address the vulnerabilities that we have identified and improve efficiency. Medicare does not pay for items or services that are not "reasonable and necessary." (Social Security Act, § 1862(a)(1)(A).) Specifically, ambulance services are covered "where the use of other methods of transportation is contraindicated by the individual's condition. . . ." (§ 1861(s)(7).) The *Medicare Benefit Policy Manual*, § 10.2.1, more specifically states that Medicare covers ambulance transports when a beneficiary's medical condition at the time of the transport is such that using other means of transportation would endanger the beneficiary's health. Coverage requirements and requirements for ambulance suppliers are in 42 CFR §§ 410.40 and 41. (OIG; OIG- 12-14-02; expected issue date: FY 2016)

Anesthesia services—Payments for personally performed services

We will review Medicare Part B claims for personally performed anesthesia services to determine whether they were supported in accordance with Medicare requirements. We will also determine whether Medicare payments for anesthesia services reported on a claim with the "AA" service code modifier met Medicare requirements. Physicians report the appropriate anesthesia modifier code to denote whether the service was personally performed or medically directed. (CMS, *Medicare Claims Processing Manual*, Pub. No. 100-04, ch. 12, § 50) Reporting an incorrect service code modifier on the claim as if services were personally performed by an anesthesiologist when they were not will result in Medicare's paying a higher amount. The service code "AA" modifier is used for anesthesia services personally performed by an anesthesiologist, whereas the QK modifier limits payment to 50 percent of the Medicare-allowed amount for personally performed services claimed with the AA modifier. Payments to any service provider are precluded unless the provider has furnished the information necessary to determine the amounts due. (Social Security Act, §1833(e).)

(OAS; W-00-13-35706; W-00-14-35706; W-00-15-35706; various reviews; expected issue date: FY 2015)

Chiropractic services—Part B payments for noncovered services

We will review Medicare Part B payments for chiropractic services to determine whether such payments were claimed in accordance with Medicare requirements. Prior OIG work identified inappropriate payments for chiropractic services furnished during calendar year (CY) 2006. Subsequent OIG work (CY 2013) also identified unallowable Medicare payments for chiropractic services. Part B pays only for a chiropractor's manual manipulation of the spine to correct a subluxation if there is a neuro-musculoskeletal condition for which such manipulation is appropriate treatment. (42 CFR § 410.21(b).) Chiropractic maintenance therapy is not considered to be medically reasonable or necessary and is therefore not payable. (CMS's *Medicare Benefit Policy Manual*, Pub. No. 100-02, ch. 15, § 30.5B.) Medicare will not pay for items or services that are not "reasonable and necessary." (Social Security Act, § 1862(a)(1)(A).) (OAS; W-00-12-35606; W-00-13-35606; W-00-14-35606; various reviews; expected issue date: FY 2015)

Chiropractic services—Questionable billing

We will determine and describe the extent of questionable billing for chiropractic services. Previous OIG work has demonstrated a history of vulnerabilities relative to inappropriate payments for chiropractic services, including recent work that identified a chiropractor with a 93-percent claim error rate and inappropriate Medicare payments of about $700,000. Although chiropractors may submit claims for any number of services, Medicare reimburses claims only for manual manipulations or treatment of subluxations of the spine that provides "a reasonable expectation of recovery or improvement of function." (CMS's *Medicare Benefit Policy Manual*, Pub. No. 100 02, ch. 15, § 240.1.3.) (OEI; 01-14-00200; expected issue date: FY 2015)

Chiropractic services—Portfolio report on Medicare Part B payments

We will compile the results of prior OIG audits, evaluations, and investigations of chiropractic services paid by Medicare to identify trends in payment, compliance, and fraud vulnerabilities and offer recommendations to improve detected vulnerabilities. Prior OIG work identified inappropriate payments for chiropractic services that were medically unnecessary, were not documented in accordance with Medicare requirements, or were fraudulent. Medicare does not pay for items or services that are not "reasonable and necessary." (Social Security Act, § 1862(a)(1)(A).) Part B pays only for a chiropractor's manual manipulation of the spine to correct a subluxation if there is a neuro-musculoskeletal condition for which such manipulation is appropriate treatment. (42 CFR § 410.21(b).) CMS's *Medicare Benefit Policy Manual*,

Pub. No. 100-02, ch. 15, § 30.5, states that chiropractic maintenance therapy is not considered to be medically reasonable or necessary and is therefore not payable. Further, § 240.1.2 of the manual establishes Medicare requirements for documenting chiropractic services. This planned work will offer recommendations to reduce Medicare chiropractic vulnerabilities detected in prior OIG work. (OAS; OIG-12-14-03; expected issue date: FY 2015)

Diagnostic radiology—Medical necessity of high-cost tests

We will review Medicare payments for high-cost diagnostic radiology tests to determine whether the tests were medically necessary and to determine the extent to which use has increased for these tests. Medicare will not pay for items or services that are not "reasonable and necessary." (Social Security Act, § 1862 (a)(1)(A).) (OAS; W-00-13-35454; W-00-14-35454; various reviews; expected issue date: FY 2015)

Imaging services—Payments for practice expenses

We will review Medicare Part B payments for imaging services to determine whether they reflect the expenses incurred and whether the utilization rates reflect industry practices. For selected imaging services, we will focus on the practice expense components, including the equipment utilization rate. Practice expenses may include office rent, wages, and equipment. Physicians are paid for services pursuant to the Medicare physician fee schedule, which covers the major categories of costs, including the physician professional cost component, malpractice insurance costs, and practice expenses. (Social Security Act, § 1848(c)(1)(B).) (OAS; W-00-13-35219; W-00-14-35219; various reviews; expected issue date: FY 2015)

Selected independent clinical laboratory billing requirements (new)

We will review Medicare payments to independent clinical laboratories to determine laboratories' compliance with selected billing requirements. We will use the results of these reviews to identify clinical laboratories that routinely submit improper claims and recommend recovery of overpayments. Prior OIG audits, investigations, and inspections have identified independent clinical laboratory areas at risk for noncompliance with Medicare billing requirements. Payments to service providers are precluded unless the provider has and furnishes upon request the information necessary to determine the amounts due. (Social Security Act, §1833(e).) We will focus on independent clinical laboratories with claims that may be at risk for overpayments. (OAS; W-00-14- 35726; W-00-15-35726; various reviews; expected issue date: FY 2015)

Ophthalmologists—Inappropriate and questionable billing

We will review Medicare claims data to identify potentially inappropriate and questionable billing for ophthalmology services during 2012. We will also determine the locations and specialties of providers with questionable billing. Medicare payments for Part B physician services, which include ophthalmologists, are authorized by the Social Security Act, § 1832(a)(1), and 42 CFR § 410.20. In 2010, Medicare allowed more than $6.8 billion for services provided by ophthalmologists. (OEI; 04-12-00280; 04-12-00281; expected issue date: FY 2015)

Physicians—Place-of-service coding errors

We will review physicians' coding on Medicare Part B claims for services performed in ASCs and hospital outpatient departments to determine whether they properly coded the places of service. Prior OIG reviews determined that physicians did not always correctly code nonfacility places of service on Part B claims submitted to and paid by Medicare contractors. Federal regulations provide for different levels of payments to physicians depending on where services are performed. (42 CFR § 414.32.) Medicare pays a physician a higher amount when a service is performed in a nonfacility setting, such as a physician's office, than it does when the service is performed in a hospital outpatient department or, with certain exceptions, in an ASC. (OAS; W-00-13-35113; W-00-14-35113; various reviews; expected issue date: FY 2015)

Physical therapists—High use of outpatient physical therapy services

We will review outpatient physical therapy services provided by independent therapists to determine whether they were in compliance with Medicare reimbursement regulations. Prior OIG work found that claims for therapy services provided by independent physical therapists were not reasonable or were not properly documented or that the therapy services were not medically necessary. Our focus is on independent therapists who have a high utilization rate for outpatient physical therapy services. Medicare will not pay for items or services that are not "reasonable and necessary." (Social Security Act, § 1862(a)(1)(A).) Documentation requirements for therapy services are in CMS's *Medicare Benefit Policy Manual*, Pub. No. 100-02, ch. 15, § 220.3. (OAS; W-00-11-35220; W-00-12-35220; W-00-13-35220; W-00-14-35220; W-00-15-35220; various reviews; expected issue date: FY 2015)

Portable x-ray equipment—Supplier compliance with transportation and setup fee requirements

We will review Medicare payments for portable x-ray equipment services to determine whether payments were correct and were supported by documentation. We will also assess the qualifications of the technologists who performed the services. Prior OIG work found that Medicare may have improperly paid portable x-ray suppliers for return trips to nursing facilities (i.e., multiple trips to a facility in 1 day). Medicare generally reimburses for portable x-ray services if the conditions for coverage are met. (42 CFR §§ 486.100–486.110.) (OAS; W-00-14-35464; various reviews; expected issue date: FY 2015)

Sleep disorder clinics—High use of sleep-testing procedures

We will examine Medicare payments to physicians, hospital outpatient departments, and independent diagnostic testing facilities for sleep-testing procedures to assess the appropriateness of Medicare payments for high-use sleep-testing procedures and determine whether they were in accordance with Medicare requirements. An OIG analysis of CY 2010 Medicare payments for Current Procedural Terminology[1] codes 95810 and 95811, which totaled approximately $415 million, showed high utilization associated with these sleep-testing procedures. Medicare will not pay for items or services that are not "reasonable and necessary." (Social Security Act, § 1862(a)(1)(A).) To the extent that repeated diagnostic testing is performed on the same beneficiary and the prior test results are still pertinent, repeated tests may not be reasonable and necessary. Requirements for coverage of sleep tests under Part B are in CMS's *Medicare Benefit Policy Manual*, Pub. No. 100-02, ch. 15, § 70. (OAS; W-00-10-35521; W-00-12-35521; W-00-13-35521; W-00-14-35521; various reviews; expected issue date: FY 2015)

---

[1] The five character codes and descriptions included in this document are obtained from Current Procedural Terminology (CPT®), copyright [2011] by the American Medical Association (AMA).

CPT is developed by the AMA as a listing of descriptive terms and five character identifying codes and modifiers for reporting medical services and procedures. Any use of CPT outside of this document should refer to the most current version of the Current Procedural Terminology available from AMA. Applicable FARS/DFARS apply.

CHAPTER 1

General Principles of Medical Documentation

The Documentation Guidelines provide specific criteria for billing each level of Evaluation and Management service. We use these guidelines when we audit provider records to make sure the level of service billed corresponds to the level of service documented. But few of us pay attention to the general medical records guidelines at the start of the Documentation Guidelines until a problem is identified. Sometimes, these problems come to light by way of the State Board of Medical Practice. If a patient or former staff member makes a complaint to the State Board of Medical Practice about billing or a treatment issue, the Board may review the physician's records. A managed-care payer may identify problems with records when visiting the practice to do quality assurance audits. An employer may question a physician's standard record keeping. Or, a new physician coming into the practice will notice records that may not be at the standard of care—records everyone else in the practice has taken for granted. When the quality of the medical record is questioned, these General Principles can provide guidance.

The emergence of electronic health records (EHR) changes the format of our medical records, solves some problems, and creates new ones. Practices that have an EHR may want to develop a set of procedures and protocols that meet the guidelines but take into account the different work processes involved in using an EHR.

Why Is Documentation Important?

The Guidelines tell us that the medical record is important because it facilitates the ability of the physician and other healthcare professionals to treat the patient over time and allows for communication and continuity of care among physicians and other healthcare professionals. An accurate medical record also supports accurate and timely claims review and payment, utilization review, and collection of data for research purposes.

Payers need information to support the claim submitted to them, including site of service, the medical necessity and appropriateness of the diagnostic or therapeutic services provided, and to know that the services provided are accurately reported on the claim form.

The Office Chart as a Whole

Assuming a paper record—an assumption that can be made less frequently each year—there are a few things I look at when I assess an office chart. (I'll talk about EHR records and two recent OIG reports later in the chapter.) I want to see the patient's name and one other identifier on the chart cover and on each page of the record. This identifier could be date of birth or medical records number. The practice should have a system in place to distinguish charts when two or more patients have the same name. Name alert stickers work well for this. They alert the staff member or provider who is using the chart to double check that the David Allen in front of them is the David Allen identified in the chart they are holding.

The patient's allergies should be prominently and consistently recorded in the record.

Good paper records have up-to-date medication lists and problem lists. It sounds simple, but can require an extensive amount of work in a busy practice. The medication list is a particular problem for patients who are taking multiple drugs or being seen by multiple providers. The practice needs to be confident that the dosages and frequencies of the medications on the medication list are accurate and current. Some practices combine the medication list with a prescription renewal form; others keep this as a separate document. Most charts also have a health history sheet, which not only documents pertinent past medical, family, and social history, but also allows the providers and staff to record the dates of preventive medicine services. At a glance, a provider can tell if the patient is overdue for a tetanus shot or needs a mammogram. This not only improves quality of care, but can provide a revenue boost to a practice.

Each document in the patient's chart should include his name and one other identifier, such as medical record number or date of birth. All pages in the chart should be affixed. That is, there should never be loose pages in a medical record. The best records have a consistent order to them and within each section (lab, progress notes, etc.), the documents are recorded chronologically. Reports and documents produced outside the office should be reviewed and initialed by the provider before they are filed in the chart.

A system must be in place to record telephone calls and the office response to the phone calls. Taking messages and recording office responses on post-it style notes is not effective without a system to permanently affix them to the chart.

All entries into the medical record should be dated and signed. If the signature or initials do not readily identify the signer, develop and use a master signature sheet. Type the name of every employee authorized to enter data into medical records. Have two date columns: date started working at the practice and date left the practice (if no longer there). Ask each staff person to initial/sign the log in her usual style and date the signature. All entries into an EHR need to be signed with the identity of the staff member. This information may be missing in the history of the present illness. I discuss that scenario later in the chapter.

The goal in this record keeping is identified in the Documentation Guidelines. All bolded sections that follow are from the Documentation Guidelines.

The medical record facilitates:
- **The ability of the physician and other health care professionals to evaluate and plan the patient's immediate treatment, and to monitor his/her health care over time; and**
- **Communication and continuity of care among physicians and other health care professionals involved in the patient's care.**

In other words, the care of the patient should not rely only on the physician's memory of that patient, but on the recording of facts, findings, diagnoses, and previous treatments documented in the record. Should that physician be on vacation, leave the practice, or retire, another physician or provider should be able to take over the care of the patient using the patient chart as the source of information.

Individual encounters in the medical record also are discussed in the General Principles section of the Documentation Guidelines. They are applicable to all types of medical and surgical services in all settings. The examples in this section relate to office records, but these guidelines serve as overarching criteria for documenting all encounters with patients.

The first principle is one that we all agree with but don't always comply with.

The medical record should be complete and legible.

Handwritten notes in the office note or hospital progress notes continue to be a problem for some physicians and providers. Handwritten notes present several problems, including legibility. If the note is not legible, no payer will consider it a reimbursable service. In addition, no one will deny the importance to patient care of notes that can be read by the provider, by the staff when the provider is away, and by other physicians and providers who participate in the care of the patient. Also, as the day wears on and additional patients are seen, the physician documents less and the handwritten notes get shorter. This affects both the quality of the record and the level of service that can be billed. Physicians who handwrite their notes rarely take the time to document all of the negative responses in the Review of Systems or all of the negative exam elements in the physical exam.

Remind physicians that legibility means more than the ability of their own partners and staff to read their writing. The note should be legible to caregivers and reviewers outside the practice as well.

If you have a provider whose handwriting is difficult to read, your practice should implement a policy to test legibility.

- The reader should be able to read along a line of writing at a regular pace. Even if every word is not decipherable, the reader should be able to understand enough to make the whole intelligible.
- If the reader needs to decipher each word, the record is not legible.
- If the clinician cannot read back his own writing after a period of time, the record is not legible.
- If healthcare professionals who do not regularly work with the clinician cannot read the record, it is not legible.

The documentation of each patient encounter should include:
- **Reason for the encounter and relevant history, physical examination findings and prior diagnostic test results;**
- **Assessment, clinical impression or diagnosis;**
- **Plan for care; and**
- **Date and legible identity of the observer.**

This second general principle of medical record documentation covers a lot of ground. Notice that the guidelines say for *each patient encounter*. Many times, looking at the entire record, the answers to these questions are clear. This is especially true in subsequent hospital visits, when the physician is dealing with the entire medical record for the patient's stay. Sometimes, the individual subsequent visit is documented with the entire record in mind, and the individual note lacks some of the elements in the above guideline. That's why this point is important and worth repeating: for *each patient encounter.* When an auditor looks at a note, each note stands on its own.

CMS has been lenient in interpreting the requirement for the "reason for the encounter," in my opinion. Notes with reasons like, "Here for follow up on labs" or "Here for follow up of chronic problems" are accepted by many contractors. Suggest to your providers that they be as specific as possible in describing the reason for the visit. The reason cited will also serve as their chief complaint.

A physician or provider is required to document the relevant history related to the presenting problem or reason for the visit, not the entire medical history, and to document relevant physical examination findings. Some types of service require only two of three of the key components, such as established patient visits, and many visits in this category do not document any physical exam or document only a brief exam.

Any prior diagnostic test results should be noted in the medical record. These can be dictated or written into the note for the day. Many providers indicate on the lab record that diagnostic test results were reviewed by initialing and dating the review. This allows them to make a short statement in the progress note, such as, "Labs reviewed and on chart," rather than re-dictating the abnormal or normal values into the record.

Every note should indicate the assessment, clinical impressions, or diagnosis. Some subsequent hospital visits will note the assessment as A: Stable. P: As above. This leaves the reviewer scouring the history to find the patient's problems. With that documentation, there is a risk that a payer auditor will not allow it as a reportable service. In some notes documented with an EHR, the entire problem list is reproduced as the assessment, whether or not all of the problems on the list were addressed at the visit. The assessment should list the problems that were addressed during each visit and the status of each problem.

The plan for care includes diagnostic tests ordered (more about that later), medications, instructions to the patient about care at home, and what symptoms require a return visit. In some notes, the plan for care may include the doctor's thinking about the patient's care. For example, "If the test results are negative, we will proceed with. . . ." These specific instructions are useful for other covering providers and can protect the physician in terms of liability issues.

The date of the encounter and the legible identity of the provider must be documented. The Documentation Guidelines do not require a signature. However, if the note is only signed (without a typewritten spelling of the name), be sure the signature is legible. Medicare does not require that a note is signed, only that the legible identity of the provider is in the note. Some types of organizations do require a signature: RHCs and offices under the auspices of JCAHO. CMS implemented rules related to electronic signatures in EHRs.

If not documented, the rationale for ordering diagnostic and other ancillary services should be easily inferred.

In many notes, the plan is explicit: "Chest x-ray for shortness of breath," or "Hemoglobin and hematocrit to check on anemia."

However, some notes list the plan but do not mention the indication in that section of the note: CBC, Chest x-ray, EKG. When the physician or provider completes the order form, the indication is spelled out. However, few order forms become part of the patient's permanent record. In many notes, the reason for the test is clear. A patient in a certain age group who presents for a preventive medicine service will likely be referred for mammography or colonoscopy. A patient who has diabetes on her problem list will have a Hemoglobin A1C ordered. A patient with an abnormal exam finding may be referred for diagnostic testing related to the abnormal exam finding, with or without a positive history. If a clinical reviewer could infer the reason for the test by reviewing the history or exam documented in the note, there is no need to re-document the indication in the plan. However, if there is any doubt, document the indication for the diagnostic or ancillary service in the plan, with the order.

Past and present diagnoses should be accessible to the treating and/or consulting physician.

An up-to-date problem list is the best tool to meet this requirement. It is inefficient for the provider to page through old medical records at each visit to find past and current diagnoses. However, the guidelines do not require any specific format; they simply say that the diagnoses should be accessible to the treating and/or consulting physician.

Appropriate health risk factors should be identified.

Health risks can be identified as they relate to the individual visit or to the patient's entire health and medical record. For example, the smoking history for a patient who presents with bronchitis is relevant for that visit. The patient's family history of Type 1 diabetes is relevant to the entire record and will likely be addressed at each preventive medicine visit.

This information should be documented in the note for the visit or in an easily accessible section of the chart that addresses the patient's own health risk factors and genetic, family risk factors. When relevant to the day's visit, the physician or provider can indicate that the health risk factors were reviewed.

The patient's progress, response to and changes in treatment, and revision of diagnosis should be documented.

This guideline is usually accomplished in several areas of the note. The history of the present illness and review of systems may document the patient's symptoms or response to treatment. The physical exam findings and lab results will also document the patient's progress. Any changes in treatment plan, medications, dosages, and recommendations should be documented in the plan section of the note for that date.

The procedural and ICD-9-CM codes reported on the health insurance claim form or billing statement should be supported by the documentation in the medical record.

Many audit sheets in this book will allow you to review your compliance with this recommendation. You can audit for level of code using the Evaluation and Management (E/M) level of service auditing tools. If you are billing for consults, critical care, or new patient visits, there are audit sheets for those specific services as well.

As part of your annual auditing and compliance program, ensuring that the CPT® and ICD-9-CM codes reported on the health insurance claim form are supported by the documentation in the medical record is key. In fact, it simply is what we do in compliance.

Many diagnosis code errors are caused by—and can be corrected by solving—two problems: 1) not understanding the conventions and guidelines for use of ICD-9 codes and 2) not coding to the highest degree of specificity.

Physician offices have been too complaisant about non-specific diagnosis coding because claims are paid with non-specific codes. Now, however, some groups with risk contracts find that using the non-specific codes can adversely affect their reimbursement. Groups that hope to participate in Accountable Care Organization projects must code underlying medical conditions accurately. And, as we prepare for ICD-10 in 2015, specificity in diagnosis coding will become critical.

Changes Due to Electronic Health Records

The format of medical records has changed from paper to electronic in many offices, and the pace of adoption of EHRs increased with the stimulus money for meaningful use. This changes the work processes for seeing a patient, storing information, and accessing information. It also changes the look of the printed note. Using an EHR does not change the provider's duty to comply with these basic medical record guidelines, but will certainly change how the work is done and what the record looks like afterwards.

Some issues become non-issues with EHR. For example, legibility is no longer an issue. The medical record is no longer stored in a single place, locked in an office at night when a treating physician may need access. Off-site access to authorized users allows on-call physicians to obtain history, problem, and medication lists.

All entries into the record still need to be signed. Some systems make it difficult to tell who documented the history of the present illness (HPI). Only the billing provider may document the HPI and the system should allow the medical assistant or nurse to sign his portion of the HPI.

The quality of the EHR notes varies widely, with some systems heavily reliant on check offs and templates that sometimes make it difficult to assess the reason for the encounter, the patient's progress, or response to treatment. In some systems, the entire problem list is entered into the assessment section. This makes it difficult to know what specific problems were addressed at this visit. The problem list is past medical history; the assessment should list only those problems that were addressed at the visit and the status of these problems.

Many systems allow easy access to past medical history, family history, and risk factors. The clinician can review these without the need for re-documentation, indicate that they were reviewed and updated, and note changes, if any.

Likewise, if the rationale for ordering the test is not easily inferred, the provider should discuss that in the assessment and plan portion of the note.

Many EHR programs have significantly improved the templates they use to document visits. Whereas the early notes often read like checklists, the more recent notes I have reviewed make it easier for the auditor (and presumably the next provider) to understand what happened at the visit. But, watch for the appearance of cloned or identical notes. The OIG is in the process of reviewing E/M notes for identical notes. These happen because a clinician copies and pastes from one visit to the next, uses a template without adding additional clinical information into the note, or pre-populates the documentation before the patient is seen. All of these instances should be avoided.

And although out of the scope of this chapter and book, using an EHR requires knowledge of and compliance with security and HIPAA standards. Electronic health records do create new problems related to the integrity of the medical record, and this was highlighted in two recent OIG reports, and noted in the popular press.

Certain medical stories are irresistible to the popular press: International Classification of Diseases, 10th edition (ICD-10) external cause codes that are ridiculous (W61.43XD, pecked by a turkey, subsequent encounter) or medical practices using their electronic health records (EHRs) in a way that increases their revenue. A recent headline was eye-catching, as headlines are meant to be: "Report finds more flaws in digitizing patient files." *The New York Times* reported on January 8, 2014. In this article, the Office of Inspector General (OIG) found Medicare and its contractors weren't doing enough to prevent fraud caused by using an electronic health record. It makes for good copy, doesn't it? (OIE-01-11-00571, CMS and its Contractors Have Adopted Few Program Integrity Practices to Address Vulnerabilities in EHRs, January 2014). It followed a December report about safeguards in hospital EHRs. (OIE-01-11-00570, Not all Recommended Fraud Safeguards Have Been Implemented in Hospital EHR Technology). Taken together, physician practices and hospitals are given fair warning about government concerns.

The December report about safeguards is a report that information technology (IT) staff, practice managers, and medical directors should review. It relates to audit functions within the EHR. (Don't go to sleep on me here.) It also had a bombshell about E/M services. The report found a lack of safeguards and issued recommendations about tracking alterations or changes to documentation. It recommended that EHRs track method of input, including copy and paste, direct entry, or import for any update. It states that EHR systems should have user authorization and access controls that positively identify by National Provider Identifier (NPI) the author of entries and restrict unauthorized access by user ID and passwords. There were other recommendations related to data transfer standards.

This same report recommended that EHR technology not prompt a user to add documentation for E/M coding but be able to alert a user to "inconsistencies between documentation and coding." There are two parts to this. First, the program shouldn't prompt the user to encourage higher codes. "Just add family history, and the visit is a 99204." The second suggests, however, that the program could warn a clinician who is coding a service at a higher level than documented.

The January report (CMS and its Contractors Have Adopted Few Program Integrity Practices to Address Vulnerabilities in EHRs) directly discusses using copy and paste and over-documentation. Quoting from the OIG report is the following:

Copy-Pasting. Copy-pasting, also known as cloning, enables users to select information from one source and replicate it in another location. When doctors, nurses, or other clinicians copy-paste information but fail to update it or ensure accuracy, inaccurate information may enter the patient's medical record and inappropriate charges may be billed to patients and third-party health care payers. Furthermore, inappropriate copy-pasting could facilitate attempts to inflate claims and duplicate or create fraudulent claims.

Over-documentation. Over-documentation is the practice of inserting false or irrelevant documentation to create the appearance of support for billing higher-level services. Some EHR technologies auto-populate fields when using templates built into the system. Other systems generate extensive documentation on the basis of a single click of a checkbox, which if not appropriately edited by the provider may be inaccurate. Such features can produce information suggesting the practitioner performed more comprehensive services than were actually rendered.

The Documentation Guidelines that we use to audit E/M services were written in 1995 and 1997, long before most groups were using an electronic health record. But they are still in place today and are the guidance we have about what parts of a previous visit can be reviewed, updated, and used in a current visit and count toward today's documentation. Here is what they say:

A ROS and/or a PFSH obtained during an earlier encounter does not need to be re-recorded if there is evidence that the physician reviewed and updated the previous information. This may occur when a physician updates his or her own record or in an institutional setting or group practice where many physicians use a common record. The review and update may be documented by:

- *describing any new ROS and/or PFSH information or noting there has been no change in the information; and*
- *noting the date and location of the earlier ROS and/or PFSH.*

Auditors and payers will allow the review of systems (ROS) and past medical, family and social history from a previous visit to be included as part of the current visit as long as the physician notes any new changes or the absence of changes. The clinician doesn't have to redo the work and the work doesn't all have to be re-documented. In a handwritten or a dictated note, that was huge time saver. The history of present illness (HPI), exam, assessment, and plan are not allowed to be copied, reviewed and notated, "No changes required" made according to the Documentation Guidelines (Guidelines).

In a paper record, it makes perfect sense. But what about in an electronic world? Most programs allow a clinician to carry forward all or part of a note and edit it. Most auditors don't credit the HPI is copied from a previous note because according to the Guidelines, *The HPI is a chronological description of the development of the patient's present illness from the first sign and/or symptom or from the previous encounter to the present. It includes the following elements:*

- *location*
- *quality*
- *severity*
- *duration*
- *timing*
- *context*
- *modifying factors*
- *associated signs and symptoms*

We interpret that to mean a description of the patient's current symptoms, not past medical history. Since the Guidelines specifically state that the ROS and Past, Family, and Social History (PFSH) but not the HPI may be carried forward, auditors expect the HPI to change from visit to visit. Often, reading a copied HPI confuses the timeframe and is inaccurate.

But clinicians see things differently. The start of the history section is often a succinct summary of the patient's condition, which is helpful to carry forward from visit to visit, as in this example:

"HPI: Pleasant 58-year-old with a past medical history of coronary artery disease, previous acute coronary syndrome. He had bypass surgery. His last cardiac catheterization was June 2011. At that time bypass grafts were patent. The third obtuse marginal demonstrated 80 percent stenosis in the proximal third. The RCA demonstrated 100 percent proximal stenosis. The mid RCA was supplied by collaterals.

There was diffuse coronary disease. Ejection fraction was 55 percent. There was no intervention at that point in time. In November he developed recurrent chest pain. He ruled out for myocardial infarction and was discharged on metoprolol as well as imdur and he is no longer on Benicar."

The physician certainly doesn't want to re-type that and does want it at the start of the visit as a reminder for future visits and for other care providers. This seems reasonable to me, but the physician needs to add the following: "Since last seen, he reports. . . ." The physician must describe the patient's symptoms, if any, or the status of the patient's condition since the last visit.

What about the exam, assessment, and plan? The Guidelines don't allow for copying those sections. Providers tell me that opening the previous note and copying the exam into today's visit reminds them of abnormal findings. The provider then edits the exam. Use extreme caution with this until we receive Centers for Medicare and Medicaid Services (CMS) guidance. It runs the risk of falling into the categories of cloning and over-documentation. I read too many notes in which I am surprised the level of exam that was documented for a follow-up or minor problem, such as a comprehensive, eight-organ system exam for a cast change on an 8-year-old. As for the assessment and plan, if the physician is following the patient for the same problems and addresses each of them at the visit, the list won't change. It's possible the status of these won't change or the treatment plan. The clinician needs to be sure to include in the list only those problems addressed that day and scrupulously update the status of them. Again, the Guidelines, themselves written in a pre-EHR era, do not allow for using and updating a previous assessment and plan.

Some clinicians complain they can't trust the information in EHR notes from another provider. The first duty in documenting a service is to the integrity and accuracy of the medical record. But keep in mind that the payer isn't paying you twice for the same work. Some notes are copied wholesale from a previous visit with minimal changes. It makes it difficult to validate the medical necessity for the service and to know what happened at the subsequent visit.

More than a little irony is in the situation. First, CMS all but insists that physicians use an electronic health record. But CMS seems to say, "Don't use this tool in a way that is too convenient or that saves you any time." Until we receive CMS guidance, while working within the constraints of the EHR, document in a manner will help you and other clinicians to treat the patient.

WHY DOES THE OIG CARE?

The Office of Inspector General (OIG) cares about these issues because they are protecting Medicare beneficiaries and taxpayer dollars. Here are the items I think are key in these General Principles:

- Legibility and identity of the provider. Be careful of hospital records that are handwritten. Suggest that the physician print or stamp her name.
- Reason for the encounter. Don't make the auditor guess.
- Indication for diagnostic tests. Since Medicare and most payers have specific indications for many diagnostic tests, the record should support those indications.
- Ability of another clinician to treat from the record. This is addressed in legibility, completeness, the requirement for current and past medical problems, and the need for the health risks to be identified. Most clinicians understand that although they have produced the medical record, they have paid for the paper on which it is printed, and their staff member files and stores the record, the information in the record belongs to the patient. And the purpose of the record exceeds the requirement that they can treat the patient from the record. The record must be useful to covering and consulting physicians.
- The medical record must support the CPT® and ICD-9-CM codes reported on the claim form. Again, this seems basic and it is. But it is the backbone of all payer requirements for the accuracy of the medical record.
- Notes that are overly templated or have large portions copied from a previous note do not provide clinical detail to other health care professionals who will treat the patient.

RED FLAGS

Auditing a sampling of medical records using the audit sheets in this section is your best warning system to determine if you have problems in the area of General Principles of documentation. That will provide a systematic review of each provider in the key areas defined by CMS. However, here are some other warning signs:

- Complaints from staff, pharmacies, or other medical offices that a note is illegible.

- Identical notes from one patient to another or one visit to another.
- Copying and pasting large portions of the note.
- Medical necessity denials for ancillary or diagnostic tests because the documentation in the medical record is not a covered diagnosis for that service.
- Notes that are significantly different than the norm. That is, when you compare the notes that your office or a particular physician produces to other medical records you receive, you find significant quality differences.
- Longstanding complaints in an office about a particular physician's documentation. Address the issue through the practice's governance process before you are required to address it by a payer or regulatory body.
- Out-of-date problem lists and medication lists. Outdated medication lists are more than a documentation problem; they affect quality of care and are a liability issue.
- Lack of a problem list or medication list.
- Incomplete health history forms on long-standing patients.
- Long, templated notes in which the reason for the visit and the assessment and plan are difficult to ascertain.
- An audit that shows that the medical record does not support the CPT® and ICD-9-CM codes billed on the claim form.
- Non-specific diagnosis coding.

COMPLIANCE RESPONSE

If you have a provider who handwrites notes and the notes are illegible, adopt EHR, hire a scribe, or use a dictation system. Illegibility puts the practice at high compliance and liability risk. Make sure the governance policies and employment agreements with physicians and other providers allow the group to address this issue—and do so. The single most risky situation in a practice is to ignore a problem that everyone knows about and acknowledges because the physician is a partner, or the founder, or a high revenue producer. Address these issues.

If notes are signed with initials or other marks that are not identifiable to those outside the practice, adopt a signature log in your procedure manual. Type the names of all providers and staff who will enter information into the medical record. Enter the dates of employment for each person and ask everyone to sign or initial the log. If asked to send a note and the signature is initialed or is a mark that is only known in your practice, send a copy of the signature log.

Document an assessment for each visit. Do not use the problem list as the assessment. Document the problems and issues that were discussed at that day's visit.

If using an electronic health record, and the history of the present illness is lacking because the provider must type it in personally, set up a system that allows the provider to dictate that part of the note. Add overdocumentation and copy/paste to your audit plan this year. When reviewing an established patient visit, review previous visits. When reviewing a subsequent hospital visit, review the initial hospital care service and other subsequent days to identify these problems.

Review templates carefully. A medical encounter documented with a series of check offs and drop down boxes still needs to reflect the nature of the encounter.

Be sure the plan for care is clear. Remind the provider that the test of clarity is not whether that provider knows what the follow-up plan is, but whether another provider, reading the chart, understands the plan of care.

Remember, there is no substitute for coding education for physicians, NPPs, and staff. Coding is complicated. Getting it right has enormous revenue and compliance implications. If you want to be sure you meet this final requirement in the General Principles of Documentation, use the Compliance Plan Audit Sheets provided on the next page:

COMPLIANCE PLAN AUDIT SHEET

Auditor Name:	Date of Audit:
Organization Name:	

General Principles of Medical Documentation – Individual Encounters

For this audit you will need the medical record for a specific encounter and the access to the entire record.

Select 10 patients per provider who have an encounter billed at any location. Complete this form for each encounter. For procedural and ICD-9-CM auditing, use other sheets in this book.

Patient ID:		Provider ID:	
DOS:	Auditor ID:	Date of Audit:	

Answer yes or no to the following questions by checking the appropriate box/circle:

Is the record legible?	❏ Yes	⭘ No
Is the encounter dated?	❏ Yes	⭘ No
Does the note indicate who provided the service?	❏ Yes	⭘ No
Is the reason for the visit documented?	❏ Yes	⭘ No
Is there a history of the present illness documented?	❏ Yes	⭘ No
Are past medical problems on the chart?	❏ Yes	⭘ No
Are the patient's current medications documented in this note or noted to be reviewed and updated on the medication list?	❏ Yes	⭘ No
If needed, is a physical exam documented?	❏ Yes	⭘ No
Are prior diagnostic results on the chart?	❏ Yes	⭘ No
Is there an assessment, clinical impression, or diagnosis?	❏ Yes	⭘ No
Is there a plan of care?	❏ Yes	⭘ No
If diagnostic tests are ordered, is the reason documented or can it be easily inferred?	❏ Yes	⭘ No
Are health risks documented?	❏ Yes	⭘ No
Are the patient's progress, response to and changes in treatment, and revision of diagnoses documented?	❏ Yes	⭘ No

COMPLIANCE PLAN AUDIT SHEET

Auditor Name:	Date of Audit:
Organization Name:	

General Principles of Medical Documentation – Medical Record as a Whole		
To perform this audit, you will need the medical record for a specific encounter and access to the entire record. Select 10 patients per provider. Complete this form for each medical record. Use this audit sheet with the encounter audit sheet.		

Patient ID:	Provider ID:		
Auditor ID:	Date of Audit:		

Answer yes or no to the following questions by checking the appropriate box/circle:

For paper charts:		
Are the patient's name and one other identifier on the chart jacket?	☐ Yes	○ No
Do all of the pages in the chart contain the patient's name and one other identifier?	☐ Yes	○ No
Are all pages attached in the record?	☐ Yes	○ No
Is the information stored in the record in the same format for each chart?	☐ Yes	○ No
Is information stored chronologically within each section?	☐ Yes	○ No
Are allergies documented prominently and in a consistent location?	☐ Yes	○ No
For all records:		
Are all entries dated and signed?	☐ Yes	○ No
Is there a completed, up-to-date problem list?	☐ Yes	○ No
Is there a completed, up-to-date medication list?	☐ Yes	○ No

CHAPTER 2

Aberrant Evaluation and Management Coding Patterns

Data mining—the words cause a chill down our backs. The Centers for Medicare & Medicaid Services (CMS) and its contractors (CERT, RAC, and MAC) have access to all paid claims data for all clinicians for all specialties, and sophisticated analysis tools. They are playing with a full deck of cards. Practices have only their own billing data and limited CMS data for comparison. Not a full deck—maybe the ace of spades and three of hearts. With CMS and its contractors selecting groups for audit based on data analysis, practices need to do what they can to compare their own data with national norms.

Aberrant Coding Patterns

An Office of Inspector General (OIG) report released in May 2012 (OIE-04-10-00180) described coding trends in Evaluation and Management (E/M) services between 2001 and 2011. The OIG noted that payments for E/M services increased by 48% during this period to $33.5 billion and that E/M services are vulnerable to fraud and abuse. The OIG found that physicians increased their level of service in all categories of code. The report showed in table and graphical format the change in codes from lower to higher levels of service. The OIG recommended that CMS continue to educate physicians in E/M coding and encouraged the Medicare administrative contractors to review billing for E/M services. CMS accepted both of these recommendations.

CMS collects data yearly by specialty of the distribution for all E/M codes; that is, how many and what percentage of each level of service in each E/M category and subcategory are billed by physicians in the aggregate. Their intermediaries statistically compare each physician and non-physician practitioner (NPP) profile against the norm for their specialty. NPPs are grouped together regardless of the specialty in which they work. It is important for practices to do this comparison for all services provided. This is commonly called the "bell curve" data, although the data are not distributed in a bell curve. Practice management systems can produce an E/M frequency report or productivity report to provide the group with the data for comparison.

It is not enough to simply audit notes using the Documentation Guidelines. It is critically important to compare the E/M profile of each provider with the norm. The norm is not meant to be prescriptive; that is, the goal is not to have every physician and NPP mimic his specialty's profile, but compare the profile and *understand* the reason for any variation.

CMS also warns us that medical necessity is the most important criterion in selecting a level of service. From Pub 100-04, Chapter 12, Section 30.6.1B :

Medical necessity of a service is the overarching criterion for payment in addition to the individual requirements of a code. It would not be medically necessary or appropriate to bill a higher level of evaluation and management service when a lower level of service is warranted. The volume of documentation should not be the primary influence upon which a specific level of service is billed. Documentation should support the level of service reported. The service should be documented during, or as soon as practicable after it is provided in order to maintain an accurate medical record.

All One Level of Service

Billing all one level of service in any category or subcategory of E/M raises red flags! Don't do it! Some providers bill all of their admissions or all of their consults at the same level. Medicare's stated policy is that medical necessity is the overarching criterion for selecting a level of service. Medicare expects that patients present with varying degrees of severity of illness and seriousness in their presenting problems, and thus the level of history and exam required for visits will vary. Billing all subsequent hospital visits or consults at one level is incorrect based on these coding policies as well as the code definitions. Providers who do this are overcoding for some services, undercoding for some services, or both. Correcting the problem may result in an increase or a decrease in revenue, but it is critically important to remedy the issue, whatever the result.

Some specialists believe they can bill all of their consults as Level 4 or Level 5 consults. I worked with a Cardiologist who began receiving pre-payment audits for his 99244 services and called me when he began receiving these requests. Unfortunately, they all audited at the 99243 level. Even more unfortunate, when I asked him, "What percentage of your consults do you bill as Level 4s?" he replied, "All of them. That's just normal for my specialty." That's not true. No specialist should bill all of their consults at one level.

All High-Level Services

When you compare your billing profile with the norm for your specialty, you may find that a physician bills many more high-level services than the CMS norm for her specialty. If so, your risk of a carrier audit increases. If this is the case, be sure to audit notes for compliance with the Documentation Guidelines for that level of service. Also, ask yourself this question: Are these patients really sicker or more complicated than the patients of other physicians of the same specialty? A Family Practitioner (FP) who treats mostly adult patients may have a profile with more high-level codes than an FP who has many young families in the practice. A subspecialist in a rural area who is the only specialist in the area may also treat disproportionately sicker patients than a subspecialist with both a primary care and a referral practice. The important thing is to look at your profile. If it is significantly different, ask yourself if the difference is justified by the type of patients and practice you have. Are you clear about the documentation requirements for the E/M services?

CMS also specifically advises carriers to warn providers about the requirements for billing high-level services. From Pub. 100-04, Ch. 12, Sec. 30.6.1D of the Medicare *Internet Only Manual*:

> **D—*Use of Highest Levels of Evaluation and Management Codes***
> *Contractors must advise physicians that to bill the highest levels of visit codes, the services furnished must meet the definition of the code (e.g., to bill a Level 5 new patient visit, the history must meet CPT®'s definition of a comprehensive history).The comprehensive history must include a review of all the systems and a complete past (medical and surgical) family and social history obtained at that visit. In the case of an established patient, it is acceptable for a physician to review the existing record and update it to reflect only changes in the patient's medical, family, and social history from the last encounter, but the physician must review the entire history for it to be considered a comprehensive history.*
>
> *The comprehensive examination may be a complete single system exam such as cardiac, respiratory, psychiatric, or a complete multi-system examination.*

Medical practices are still allowed to use the 1995 or the 1997 Documentation Guidelines. The definition of a comprehensive history and exam are found in those Guidelines.

All Low-Level Services

Billing all low-level codes does not protect a provider from an audit because the billing profile will still be different from the norm for the specialty. A government or private payer is less likely to ask for a refund for services billed at too low a level, but the goal is to submit services at the level that reflects the work performed and documented.

One issue with this coding profile is the potential for lost revenue. If you find a physician profile like this in your practice, ask yourself the same questions you asked if the profile was unusually high. Is the patient population really different from the patient population in other practices? Does the physician understand the guidelines? The coding could accurately represent the level of service performed and the documentation of the service. Perhaps this physician provides mostly a walk-in service for acute visits rather than treating a group of chronically ill patients. Those visits may cluster at lower-level visits.

Another flag to audit is billing a procedure and a low-level E/M service every time. For example, a Podiatrist visits a nursing facility and bills the lowest-level nursing visit code *with every nail treatment*. That would not be medically necessary, and using a low-level code not only does not protect from an audit, it raises a flag! The National Correct Coding Initiative chapter guidelines and the *Medicare Claims Processing Manual* both note that the decision to perform a minor procedure is included in the payment for a procedure, and billing an E/M service on the same day must meet the requirements for a separate and distinct service.

Overuse of 99211

The use of 99211, typically nurse visits, varies by specialty and practice. If your coding profile shows that your practice bills a significantly higher percentage of 99211s (as a percentage of your total established patient visits), you may want to review your billing policies and guidelines for a nurse visit. See the chapter on Billing for 99211 and specific audit tools for a more detailed discussion.

No Visits in a Category or Subcategory

If you run your report and find that some providers have no services billed in a category or subcategory, ask yourself if that is correct and accurate. For example, does your practice have no new patients but many consults? Are all of the patients who present to the practice for the first time considered consults, or are some of those visits really new patients?

Remember that Medicare stopped recognizing consultation codes in 2010, but many private payers continue to accept these codes. If you know that your providers see patients in the Emergency Department (ED) but no ED visits are billed, again, ask yourself if the practice is billing consults or outpatient visits when the actual service provided is an ED visit. Observation services are a huge source of confusion for physicians. If no observation services are billed but you believe your physicians may have admitted patients to observation status at the hospital, research this area.

Some third-party payers have audited consults and found some visits were billed as consults although they did not meet the criteria and some consults were billed at a higher level than documented. See the chapter on Consultations for more details. Errors also exist in new patient versus established patient visit codes.

New patients pay better than established patients. A large, multi-location group received a letter from a contractor asking the practice to perform a self-audit of its new patient visits. Practices with multiple locations, multiple providers, and multiple specialties are more likely to have new patient/established patient visit code errors. Some of these errors are the result of lack of understanding of what constitutes a new patient; some may be the result of a computer system or medical records system that does not allow providers to easily access this information. Decentralized medical records or a computer system that purges procedure history data in fewer than three years can make researching the new vs. established patient questions more difficult. See the New Patient Visits chapter for more information and audit sheets.

Billing hospital services can also be the source of category errors. For example, physicians may bill critical care services when the patient is not critically ill; a hospital visit initial service or subsequent hospital visit is the accurate code to bill. Critical care is a highly reimbursed service and the carrier regularly asks for notes to validate the patient's status and that time was documented in the medical record. See the chapter on Critical Care services for more information on billing and auditing critical care services.

WHY DOES THE OIG CARE?

The Office of Inspector General (OIG) cares about level of service for a number of reasons: Its sampling and auditing tells investigators that this is an area of high error rate, errors cost the program money, and the guidelines are confusing. Small changes in the physician profile translate into large sums of money for the government. The May 2012 OIG report on trends in E/M coding noted the high dollar value of Part B payments for E/M services and the change from billing lower-level codes to higher-level codes between 2001 and 2010. The OIG also noted that this was the first in a series of reports about E/M services.

According to the Comprehensive Error Rate Testing (CERT) data, specific types of services have higher error rates. For example, hospital visits have a higher error rate than established patient visits. You can check the CMS web site and find the CERT error report for services processed by your carrier.

The government also is interested in the reliability and validity of codes. If Medicare pays for a Level 3 new patient visit in California and a Level 3 new patient visit in Kentucky, it wants to be sure it's paying for the same service. The OIG wants the use of codes to be valid, i.e., the service provided is accurately described by the code billed. The OIG also wants the use of the codes to be reliable, i.e., the correct code for the service is billed every time. This is easier when the definition of the code is clear and concise. No one would say that the definitions of the E/M codes as described by either set of Documentation Guidelines are clear and concise!

There is also the potential for error in the selection of the category or subcategory of code. Selecting the correct category of E/M code often can be the most challenging issue for clinicians.

The OIG cares because E/M services, in their words, are "vulnerable to abuse."

RED FLAGS

Every practice should examine the E/M profile for each provider regularly. A 6- or 12-month period provides a good sample size. If you have educated physicians and NPPs, performed an audit, or have some reason to think the profile might have changed, re-run the report.

If you find any of the following, there is reason for concern:

- All of one level of service in any category or subcategory.
- An E/M profile that is significantly different from your specialty's national average.
- Too many low-level codes.
- All high-level codes.
- An unusual number of nurse visits (99211) for your specialty.
- Stated lack of understanding on the part of providers.
- An audit history of incongruence between billed and audited level.

- High-level visits billed when the presenting problem is straightforward.
- A significant change in profile after implementing an electronic health record.

COMPLIANCE RESPONSE

Compare every provider's E/M coding distribution to the specialty's norms twice per year. Compare the profiles, analyze variances, and address issues. At the same time, be sure to look at category and subcategory of E/M services, particularly in the area of consults, new patient visits, and critical care. These are areas that have frequent errors and significant reimbursement implications, and are areas of government interest.

The result of your analysis may lead you to audit your E/M services for level of service. Many practices do this annually. It is particularly important to do an audit annually if your previous year's results showed a high error rate for any provider or in any category of service, or if an analysis of the category or subcategory billing is unusual.

Focus your E/M auditing on providers and areas that seem high-risk. Some practices vary the category of service they audit from year to year; for example, office visits one year, hospital visits another. This can help you identify problem areas and solve them more effectively. This is a good way to use your limited compliance resources.

COMPLIANCE PLAN AUDIT SHEET

Auditor Name:	Date of Audit:
Organization Name:	

Aberrant Evaluation and Management Coding Patterns		
For this audit, run a report of your E/M coding distribution for all providers in your practice for a 6- or a 12-month period.		
Provider ID:		
DOS:	Auditor ID:	Date of Audit:

Answer yes or no to the following questions by checking the appropriate box/circle:

Does the provider bill all of any one category or subcategory of service at one level?	☐ Yes	○ No
Is the E/M profile significantly different from the national profile for your specialty?	☐ Yes	○ No
Does the provider bill at the highest two levels in all categories of codes greater than 85% of the time?	☐ Yes	○ No
Is there an unusually high percentage of 99211s for your specialty?	☐ Yes	○ No
Does the provider express confusion about coding for the level of service?	☐ Yes	○ No
Did the provider have a greater than 20% error rate on last year's audit?	☐ Yes	○ No

Count the boxes (☐ Yes) that you checked.	
0-3 ☐ Yes Checks	Address the areas of confusion or error with the provider.
4-5 ☐ Yes Checks	Include provider in this area in your compliance activities this year.
6-8 ☐ Yes Checks	Make E/M services and categories a major priority in your compliance activity for this provider for this year.

CHAPTER 3

How to Audit Evaluation and Management Services

Take a course. Buy a book. Have an experienced auditor train you. Read Medicare's Documentation Guidelines twice over. Do not assume because you can code, you can audit. Do have an experienced auditor re-audit your notes when you start auditing. No matter what your experience level, **always** use an audit sheet. This chapter serves as a companion to these educational activities to teach you to audit; it does not serve as a substitute.

The 1995 and 1997 Documentation Guidelines can be found at the Centers for Medicare & Medicaid Services (CMS) web site at http://www.cms.gov/Outreach-and-Education/Medicare-Learning-Network-MLN/MLNEdWebGuide/EMDOC.html. This chapter will discuss how to audit Evaluation and Management (E/M) notes for the correct level of service.

The source for the definition of the E/M level of services is the CPT® book. In the E/M section of the CPT® book, each code is described as needing either two or all three of the key components of history, exam, and medical decision making. The level of history, exam, and medical decision making for each level of service is named "detailed" or "comprehensive." The Documentation Guidelines, jointly developed by CMS and the American Medical Association, describe what is needed for each type of history, exam, and medical decision making.

There are four levels of history: 1) problem focused; 2) expanded problem focused; 3) detailed; and 4) comprehensive. The four levels of exam are defined with the same labels: 1) problem focused; 2) expanded problem focused; 3) detailed; and 4) comprehensive. Medical decision making is defined by four levels as well: 1) straightforward; 2) low; 3) moderate; and 4) high. If time can be used to determine the E/M code, the typical time is also listed in the CPT® book. Time is not a factor in Emergency Department (ED) visits and most preventive medicine visits. In addition, the severity of the nature of the presenting problem, a non-key factor, is defined in CPT.

Using an Electronic Medical Record to Document E/M Services

The Documentation Guidelines were developed in 1995 and revised in 1997, long before an electronic medical record (EMR) was in common use. This chapter will discuss issues with auditing EMR-created notes throughout, but the topic deserves special attention. In 2011 (and continued in 2012) the Office of Inspector General has identified identical notes on their annual Work Plan. Here is how the Office of Inspector General (OIG) described this project then:

> We will assess the extent to which CMS made potentially inappropriate payments for E/M services and the consistency of E/M medical review determinations. We will also review multiple E/M services for the same providers and beneficiaries to identify electronic health records (EHR) documentation practices associated with potentially improper payments. Medicare contractors have noted an increased frequency of medical records with identical documentation across services. Medicare requires providers to select the code for the service based upon the content of the service and have documentation to support the level of service reported. (CMS's Medicare Claims Processing Manual, Pub. No. 100–04, ch. 12, § 30.6.1.) (OEI; 04–10–00181; 04–10–00182; expected issue date: FY 2013; work in progress)

I discussed the findings of this report in the previous chapter, detailing the OIG definition of over-documentation and copy/paste or cloning. At the end of the report, the OIG recommended that CMS develop policies related to this area of concern. CMS is currently doing so.

As auditors, we often refer to these notes as cloned notes. They are notes with excessive amounts of copying and pasting from a previous visit, or so highly templated that it is difficult to determine why the patient was seen and what occurred at the visit. The history of the present illness section of the note should describe why the patient is being seen for that day, and the patient's symptoms or complaints since the last visit. The status of the patient's chronic problems could be described in place of the history of the present illness (HPI) elements. This section of the note should never be copied from a previous visit. If the information is copied, put it in past medical history with a remark that it was reviewed. Importing a "normal" review of systems (ROS) and all of past medical, family, and social history (PFSH) in an EMR note leads to HPI/ ROS inconsistencies and notes that seem odd. Why is there a complete ROS and all of PFSH for a quick re-check or a visit billed as a 99212? It doesn't seem believable. Sometimes, less is more.

Using a "normal" exam also leads to problems in EMR-generated notes. The purpose is to save the physician or provider from too many clicks to document the exam—an admirable goal. The clinician will select "normal female exam follow-up visit" and then edit the exam portion. The problem comes when the editing is not done. A patient admitted with an MI is noted to have "gait—non-antalgic." I highly doubt the patient was asked to walk while being admitted. Or, "normal external ears" is documented on every patient, whether the chief complaint was related to ears or not. When auditing a series of notes, an auditor may find that the exact same exam is used for every visit, no matter the presenting problem. This gives the appearance of cloned or identical notes.

When auditing an assessment, it is often not clear which problems on the list were addressed at that visit. The clinician will list 6 or 8 or 18 problems, some clearly historical and not addressed at this visit. "Status post hysterectomy 1994." How the patient is doing with regard to the problems won't be noted, and the same problem list will be imported as the assessment from visit to visit. The plan is a series of statements, "All questions were answered. Plan was explained to the patient. Risks described." But the reader can't tell what the plan was.

When auditing an EMR note, the auditor often makes judgments about what to count and whether to credit certain elements that seem excessively documented. Auditors may question the necessity of the documentation when compared to the presenting problem. The EMR may have a software program that suggests a level of service to the clinician. Use caution with these unless an experienced auditor has reviewed the level of service suggested regularly and extensively; they are prone to error. Unfortunately, using an EMR to document an E/M note does not make coding or auditing any easier.

1995 or 1997 Guidelines

Should you use the 1995 or 1997 Guidelines? Currently, CMS tells us that we can audit an encounter using whichever set of Guidelines is more beneficial to the provider. Some practices decide to use one or the other exclusively, but this is their own internal policy decision. There is no requirement that a provider or practice use only one set, and the practice risks losing income by not allowing the flexibility of using whichever set is more beneficial to the provider—that is, the one that results in the higher code selection.

Auditors tend to like the 1997 Guidelines because of the greater specificity of the exam components. On the other hand, providers often respond in dismay to the "counting" in that very same exam.

Can You Mix and Match the Two Sets?

Can you use the 1995 history with the 1997 exam? This was a hotly debated topic among auditors. In September of 2013, CMS released a frequently asked question about this topic, allowing the use of the history from one set of guidelines with the exam from the other.

> **FAQ on 1995 & 1997 Documentation Guidelines for Evaluation & Management Services.**
>
> Q. Can a provider use both the 1995 and 1997 Documentation Guidelines for Evaluation and Management Services to document their choice of evaluation and management HCPCS code?
>
> A. For billing Medicare, a provider may choose either version of the documentation guidelines, not a combination of the two, to document a patient encounter. However, beginning for services performed on or after September 10, 2013 physicians may use the 1997 documentation guidelines for an extended history of present illness along with other elements from the 1995 guidelines to document an evaluation and management service.

There is a significant difference in the history of the present illness component of the 1995 and the 1997 Guidelines. To reach the level of HPI required for a detailed or comprehensive history, the 1995 Guidelines require four elements of the history of the present illness. The 1997 Guidelines allow you to use either four HPI elements or the status of three chronic diseases. This is particularly helpful for Primary Care Physicians who treat adults with multiple chronic diseases. Many of these diseases are "silent" in terms of symptoms, particularly if the patient is in good control. For example, a patient with hypertension, hyperlipidemia, and diabetes, who is in good control, may complain of no symptoms to document for the HPI. Documenting the status of these conditions is a clinically relevant alternative.

The exams are radically different in the 1995 and 1997 versions of the Guidelines. There is very little definition of the body areas or organ systems in the 1995 exam. Specifically, the difference between an expanded problem focused and a detailed exam is open to interpretation. A comprehensive, single organ system exam is not defined. I will discuss this further in the section on auditing the exam. When the 1997 Guidelines were released, the general multi-system exam was a relief to auditors, but disliked by many physicians. It is very specific and relies on counting "bullets." The 1997 Guidelines also provided single specialty exams, which were helpful and clinically relevant for many specialties.

The Nature of the Presenting Problem

One of the non-key components of an E/M service is the nature of the presenting problem. The nature of the presenting problem is described for each E/M service in the CPT® book. For example, for 99203, CPT® says, "Usually, the presenting problem(s) are of moderate severity." This does not mean moderate medical decision making. In the introductory section of the E/M codes in the CPT® book, the nature of the presenting problem is described as minimal, self-limited or minor, low, moderate, or high. These are not interchangeable with medical decision making. They are not typically included on audit sheets. Ask the clinician whether it was necessary to document a detailed history and detailed exam for a minor problem. There may be times when it *is* necessary in order to rule out a more serious condition. Consider the nature of the presenting problem in addition to medical necessity when all visits are documented and billed at a high level.

> **From the CPT® book:**
>
> A presenting problem is a disease, condition, illness, injury, symptom, sign, finding, complaint, or other reason for encounter, with or without a diagnosis being established at the time of the encounter. The E/M codes recognize five types of presenting problems that are defined as follows:
>
> **Minimal:** a problem that may not require the presence of the physician or other qualified healthcare professional, but services provided under the physician's or other qualified healthcare professional's supervision.
>
> **Self-limited or minor:** a problem that runs a definite and prescribed course, is transient in nature, and is not likely to permanently alter health status OR has a good prognosis with management/compliance.

Low severity: A problem where the risk of morbidity without treatment is low; there is little to no risk of mortality without treatment; full recovery without functional impairment is expected.

Moderate severity: A problem where the risk of morbidity without treatment is moderate; there was moderate risk of mortality without treatment; uncertain prognosis OR increased probability of prolonged functional impairment.

High severity: A problem where the risk of morbidity without treatment is high to extreme; there was a moderate to high risk of mortality without treatment OR high probability of severe, prolonged functional impairment.

Auditing the History Section of the Note

The 2011 CPT® book added new charts in the E/M section that show the nature of the presenting problem for each level of E/M service. Auditors have always considered the nature of the presenting problem, but it is not typically addressed on audit sheets. With CMS concerns about cloned notes and the level of E/M services, and CPT® adding clarification about the nature of the presenting problem, auditors should take this into account when assigning a level of service.

The history component of the Documentation Guidelines consists of four elements: chief complaint, the history of the present illness (HPI), review of systems (ROS), and past medical, family, and social history (PFSH). Some or all are required, depending on the level of service billed. To qualify for the specific level of service, all three history elements of HPI, ROS, and PFSH must be met.

The Documentation Guidelines (DG) say this about the chief complaint:

CHIEF COMPLAINT (CC): The CC is a concise statement describing the symptom, problem, condition, diagnosis, physician recommended return, or other factor that is the reason for the encounter, usually stated in the patient's words.

DG: The medical record should clearly reflect the chief complaint.

Some auditors insist that the chief complaint or reason for the visit be explicitly stated in a section labeled Chief Complaint. However, the Guidelines also say this:

DG: The CC, ROS and PFSH may be listed as separate elements of history, or they may be included in the description of the history of the present illness.

It would be incorrect to insist that the chief complaint be listed in a separate section, as long as the reason for the visit was clear from the section of the note in which the history was recorded. As long as the auditor can identify from the history the reason for the visit or the nature of the patient's presenting problems, the requirement for a chief complaint is met.

Often, the chief complaint will be the patient's own statement of the problem. "I've had a hacking cough for three days." Sometimes, the problem defines the chief complaint, "Patient is here for follow up of multiple chronic problems." The chief complaint can be inferred in the history and does not need to be in its own section labeled Chief Complaint.

The history of the present illness is defined in both sets of Guidelines (1995 and 1997) by eight specific elements. (We'll talk about the status of three chronic diseases as described by the 1997 Guidelines in the next section.) When auditing the HPI, use an audit sheet that allows you to write the symptom you are using for that category next to the element. For example, next to Location, you would write, "Arm," and next to Severity you would write, "Worse" or "Better." This will keep you from using the same symptom twice or the same element more than once. It will also be helpful if you meet with the provider in a feedback session about the results of her audit. It saves you from re-auditing the note as you work with the physician and second guessing yourself! Remind physicians to document how the patient *feels since his last visit.*

Use the chart on the next page to help you audit the HPI elements. Beside each element is a definition and typical words used to describe the element. The list is not exhaustive but gives examples of the type of words that meet the definition. Experienced auditors can audit the same HPI and find different elements. As long as each one's selection of HPI elements is supported by the documentation, both are correct.

FIGURE 1. History of the Present Illness

HISTORY OF THE PRESENT ILLNESS		
Element	How do you describe the symptoms?	Sample Words
Location	Where is the patient's pain? Where do the symptoms occur?	Chest, lung, head, stomach. Some payers require specificity: left lower quadrant, not just abdomen.
Quality	What is it like? What are the characteristics of the symptoms?	Burning, dull, sharp, green, bright, stabbing, scratchy, red
Severity	How bad are the symptoms?	Better, worse, increasing, decreasing, well, same, 5 of 10 on pain scale, BP at home shows good control
Duration	When did the symptoms start? How long has the patient had the symptoms?	Today, weeks, months, longstanding, years
Timing	When do the symptoms occur?	Upon awakening, intermittently, always, still, continuous, after meals, persistent
Content	Are the symptoms associated with any activities?	After surgery, in a motor vehicle accident, when elevated, at work
Modifying Factors	What has the patient tried to relieve the symptoms?	With ice, using meds, with OTC lotion
Associated Signs and Symptoms	What other symptoms does the patient have, associated with the presenting problem?	Fever, confused, achy, weakness, pain, fatigue, swelling

The elements of the HPI typically are positive responses. If a patient has multiple complaints, you can have one or two elements from each of two or three complaints, to total four elements. Each individual complaint does not require four elements, but the sum must be four elements. Most auditors will not credit the same element twice, although this is not in the original Guidelines. For example, a patient with wrist pain and back pain would not have two elements counted for location. This is another area in which the Guidelines do not provide a specific answer. I use each HPI element only once.

This paragraph represents *my opinion* and interpretation of the Guidelines. Can you *assume location* in a history if the word does not appear in the HPI? Like so many auditing questions, CMS does not address this question directly and so as auditors, we must rely on our own judgment. *In my opinion* you can sometimes assume location, even if the physician or non-physician practitioner does not name it in the history. For example, if the provider notes that the patient has laryngitis, I will give credit for throat for location. (Where else could it be?) If the provider notes "Patient GERD symptoms better on Prilosec," I will credit stomach for the location. I will use location when the disease or symptom is specific to the location and the location can be reasonable assumed. *This is my opinion.* No one at CMS or at any contractor has directed me to do this.

I do not give credit location for psychiatric complaints or for a complaint like dizziness. There are multiple causes of dizziness (ear, neurologic, cardiac), so I don't think it's reasonable to assume location. Here are some examples when *in my opinion* you can assume location:

FIGURE 2. Crediting Location

If a provider says:	I credit:
heavy bleeding (in a GYN note)	uterus
coughing	lung
bloody stools	rectum/bowel
laryngitis	throat
GERD symptoms	stomach
SOB	lung

This is my opinion. Many auditors will not credit a location unless you can point to it and you see it named in the HPI by the clinician.

Have an Internal Policy

Some auditors insist that all of the HPI elements relate to a single problem. If a patient comes in with a head cold and knee pain, these auditors would select one of these and find the HPI elements that relate only to it. Other auditors would allow HPI elements related to the cold *and* the knee. The Guidelines are not specific about this. I will count HPI elements for two unrelated problems.

When there are gray areas—Can you assume location? Can you use an HPI element twice?—develop an internal written policy and follow it consistently. Document your reasons for developing the policy, the clinical back up for the policy, and follow it.

Who Can Document the HPI?

Only the billing provider may document the chief complaint and the HPI components of the history. Ancillary staff may not document the HPI and have that history count as part of the documentation in support of the service level in auditing the note. Where is this written? The Documentation Guidelines explicitly state that ancillary staff may record the ROS and PFSH. The Guidelines do *not* state that the HPI may be recorded by ancillary staff. The ancillary staff member often documents the chief complaint. Since the provider typically restates the reason for the visit in the HPI, and the chief complaint is permitted to be inferred and part of the HPI, this is not a problem. It is not that we are "counting" the chief complaint that the ancillary staff recorded, but that the chief complaint is recorded in the provider's history. Providers often question this rule and want to count the HPI taken by the nurse. But it is clear that HPI elements recorded by the staff may not be counted when auditing the level of service.

Status of Three Chronic Diseases

The 1997 Guidelines allow providers to document the status of three chronic conditions instead of four elements of the HPI for a detailed or comprehensive history.

It is *not* enough to simply list the conditions in this way: The patient returns for follow up of hypertension, diabetes, and high cholesterol. The provider must describe the *status* of the chronic conditions. For example:

> **Diabetes.** *She did not bring in her blood sugars. She reports that mostly they are under good control, but when she goes off her diet her blood sugars go up. Her last hemoglobin A1c was 8.3.*

> **Osteoporosis.** *Again, she is on no calcium or other medications at her preference. She was concerned about kidney stones. She does not have hypercalcuria on a recent 24-hour urine and she should be able to tolerate a calcium supplement.*

> **Hyperlipidemia.** *She feels that the Lipitor is causing nighttime sore throat and sweats as well as daytime fatigue. She apparently stopped it a few weeks ago and the symptoms went away.*

In summary, the HPI is a description of the patient's symptoms relating to the presenting problem. The 1997 Guidelines allow us to substitute the status of three chronic diseases in place of the elements of the HPI. Listing them is insufficient.

Review of Systems

Here's how the Documentation Guidelines describe the review of systems (ROS) section of the history:

A ROS is an inventory of body systems obtained through a series of questions seeking to identify signs and/or symptoms, which the patient may be experiencing or has experienced.

ROS involves the following systems:

- Constitutional symptoms (e.g., fever, weight loss)
- Eyes
- Ears, Nose, Mouth, Throat
- Cardiovascular
- Respiratory
- Gastrointestinal
- Genitourinary
- Musculoskeletal
- Integumentary (skin and/or breast)
- Neurological
- Psychiatric
- Endocrine
- Hematologic/Lymphatic
- Allergic/Immunologic

What ROS Statements Count?

Auditors struggle with when and what to credit in the review of systems. We have heard that we cannot double dip—a phrase that always makes me want a chocolate and vanilla ice cream cone. We wonder if a statement is past medical history or review of systems. We ask ourselves if non-contributory really means negative or if it just means not asked. We implore our providers not to say "unremarkable."

When you are deciding what ROS statements are acceptable, go back to the source documents: the 1995 and 1997 Documentation Guidelines themselves. Forget what you heard at a seminar or read in a newsletter unless the Guidelines confirm the facts.

Here are some non-exhaustive examples of symptoms that describe each system. To get credit for the system, the provider must document one positive or negative item from the system.

- **Constitutional:** Fevers, chills, weight change, fatigue, general health, sweating
- **Eyes:** Wears glasses, blurry vision, eye problems, double vision, loss of vision, eye pain
- **Ears/Nose/Mouth/Throat:** Hearing loss, ringing in ears, ear aches, drainage, sinus problems, nose bleeds, bad breath, sores or bleeding in mouth, changes in voice, sore throat
- **Cardiovascular:** Chest pain, chest tightness, SOB with walking, swelling of feet or hands, palpitations
- **Respiratory:** Cough, SOB, wheezing, sputum, coughing up blood
- **GI:** Change in bowel habits, nausea, vomiting, diarrhea, constipation, belly pain, rectal bleeding
- **GU:** Frequency, pain or burning on urination, change in force when urinating, blood in urine, incontinence, pain with menstruation, change in menstrual habits, testicle pain, erectile dysfunction
- **Musculoskeletal:** Joint pain or stiffness, swelling, muscle pain, back pain, difficulty walking
- **Integumentary:** Rash, itching, change in skin color, varicose veins, breast pain, lump or swelling
- **Neurological:** Headaches, lightheadedness, dizziness, tremors, numbness or tingling, weakness, paralysis
- **Psychiatric:** Memory loss, confusion, suicidal ideation, depression, anxiety, hallucinations
- **Endocrine:** Excessive thirst or urination, heat or cold intolerance, dry skin, night sweats, hair loss, brittle nails
- **Hematologic/Lymphatic:** Bleeding or easy bruising, anemia, phlebitis, enlarged glands
- **Allergic/Immunologic:** Environmental allergies, food allergies

Does the Provider Need to Say It Twice?

There is no requirement in the Guidelines that tell us that the provider must restate symptoms in a system in a separate ROS section of the note if she has documented those symptoms in the HPI. That is, if the patient comes in with a GI complaint, and the provider has documented these symptoms in the HPI, the provider does not need to re-document the GI system in the ROS section of the note to get credit for the GI system.

Some auditors will never count the system described as the chief symptom in the HPI as a system reviewed in the ROS. They consider that "double dipping." There is no official citation in support of this. If a physician has reviewed a system in describing the patient's symptoms in the HPI, I credit it in the ROS. *That is my opinion.* Each auditor or physician group should develop a policy about this and follow it consistently.

Review of Systems Statements

Past medical history is not ROS. If a physician says, "No history of hypertension," that is PMH. A review of systems for Cardiology might read, "No history of chest pain, palpitations, dyspnea on exertion," or simply, "No cardiac symptoms." Either of the last two statements shows that the clinician asked about the patient's symptoms, not just the history.

Positive systems and pertinent negative systems related to the presenting problem must be documented explicitly. That is, name the system and document the symptoms or the absence of symptoms for any system related to the patient's complaint or reason for the visit. After that, if a complete systems review was obtained, a provider may say, "Except as above, all other systems were reviewed and are negative."

Here are some **documentation examples** of what counts as a complete ROS, *after* all positives are noted and pertinent negatives are listed:

"Except as above, all other systems were reviewed and are negative."

"An extensive review of systems was obtained and except as listed in the HPI, all others are negative."

"All other systems are negative." (Better: "All other systems are reviewed and are negative.")

Here are some examples of ROS statements that *do not* meet the criteria for a complete ROS:

"ROS is unremarkable."

"ROS otherwise unremarkable."

"The ROS is non-contributory."

"ROS—negative."

After a brief HPI, "ROS—all else negative." No other pertinent negatives are specifically documented.

None of the above statements clarifies that the provider did a complete system review and found the patient's responses to be negative. It would be incorrect to give the provider credit for these vague statements.

All Others Negative

The last example addresses the issue of the requirement to document *pertinent negatives relating to the presenting problem specifically.* This requirement often trips up providers. They attend a coding course and hear the magic words "All others negative," and do not remember that in order for that to count as a complete ROS, they must document the positive systems and explicitly document negatives related to the presenting problem or affected organ system.

For example, a patient presents with a cough. The physician reviews the respiratory system and then states, "Remainder of ROS negative," and expects to get credit for a complete ROS. However, for a patient with a cough, you might expect these pertinent systems to be explicitly documented: Constitutional (fevers, chills); ENT (post nasal drip, congestion, sore throat); GI (reflux symptoms, nausea/vomiting); and Musculoskeletal (aches). If the physician reviewed those systems and they were all negative, the physician could say, "Constitutional, ENT, GI, and MS systems reviewed and all negative." Then, the physician is permitted to say, "All others negative" and get credit for a complete ROS. But remember, the physician must ask about at least ten systems in order to be credited with a complete ROS.

Unremarkable and Non-Contributory

What about "ROS otherwise unremarkable?" Can you count this toward a complete ROS? No. First, specific negatives must be documented. Second, what does "unremarkable" mean? Were all systems queried by the physician? Were there positives that weren't related to the presenting problem that are not documented? Some contractors have specifically stated that unremarkable is not acceptable. I never credit all systems for "unremarkable."

Non-contributory carries the same problem as unremarkable. The auditor has no way of knowing if the questions were asked, were asked and were negative, or were asked and were positive but do not contribute to the current illness. Do not give credit.

Forms and Staff Members

Either the patient or an ancillary staff member may fill out a form that documents past medical history, family and social history, and ROS as long as there is evidence that the provider reviewed the information. For this form to be counted as part of the documentation for a particular day, the billing provider must tie it to the day's visit. The provider must confirm that the information was reviewed. A statement such as, "The patient's ROS and PFSH, completed on the health history form, were reviewed with the patient today." It is a good practice if the provider notes something from the form. "Her ROS is positive for depression and persistent skin rashes." The provider could also sign and date the form. Sometimes I see that the provider has added more detail to the information included on the form. In an EMR, that form may be scanned into the chart or the information entered by a staff member.

Also, an ROS or PFSH documented at a previous encounter does not need to be re-recorded, as long as there is evidence that the physician or provider reviewed it and noted any changes. The date and location of the previous history must be documented. An example of this statement is, "The ROS and PFSH done here on Jan. 19, 2012 were reviewed and are unchanged except for the following. . . ." If a patient has completed a health history form, it is useful if the form has a place for the provider to sign and date, indicating that the information was reviewed. Give the reference to the original note at which the history was obtained. Reviewing the previously recorded ROS does not give a provider credit for a ROS on a subsequent visit unless the questions are re-asked of the patient.

Physicians should not simply say, "Past medical history reviewed." Tell us what you reviewed, if there were changes, and the date and location of the previous history.

What about copying and pasting from a previous note documented in an electronic health record? I strongly advise against doing that for the review of systems. The ROS is used to describe today's symptoms. There is too high a risk of the HPI and the ROS contradicting one another when an ROS from a previous note is copied and brought forward. The Guidelines allow us to use the previous ROS *only if* the physician reviews it with the patient. If the staff member drops it into the note, that is not the same as the physician reviewing it with the patient.

Templates and Contradictions

Whether using a paper form or an EMR, using templates can create problems. There can be HPI/ROS contradictions. The HPI can be documented with just checks or single words, which makes it difficult to understand why the patient presented today. The importance of the HPI is to tell the story about why the patient came for a visit and the issues and concerns the patient noted. Too much templating makes that difficult to ascertain. Similarly, if the HPI says one thing but the ROS says something else, an auditor will question all of the parts of the note that appear to be copied. A payer auditor may request notes from a previous visit to see how much of the two notes is exactly the same.

Past Medical, Family, and Social History (PFSH)

The patient's past medical history includes medications, chronic illnesses, resolved illnesses, past surgical history, and past medical treatment.

To meet the requirement of documenting the past medical history, the provider does not need to document the patient's entire past medical history in detail. The provider should document the past medical history as it is relevant to that day's visit. For some office visits, that will involve a listing of medications and allergies and a statement of current medical problems treated. For more extensive visits, such as admissions and consults, a more complete past medical history may be clinically relevant. The guidelines do not prescribe how much of the patient's past medical history needs to be described—that is left to the clinician's discretion.

The patient's family history describes a review of the medical history of the patient's family—in particular, diseases that can be hereditary or increase the patient's risk. Many high-level notes that I audit, such as initial hospital services or consults, meet all other criteria for that level of service but lack family history. Providers sometimes believe it is irrelevant to the patient's presenting problem or illness or injury.

However, if the Guidelines require family history for that particular level of service, it must be documented. Some providers say, "Family history—non-contributory." A few contractors have said they will not count "non-contributory" for family history. It carries the same problem in this section as it did in the ROS section. I recommend that the provider either document the family history or write "The patient's family history was reviewed and there is no history of *cardiac disease* or *cancer* or *neurological disorders.*" A surgeon might say, "Patient's family history is negative for bleeding disorder." The provider should be clear that the family history was reviewed. "Family history reviewed, not pertinent to today's visit." Contractors will vary in how they credit that statement. The best course is to document the patient's family medical history for all high-level visits for which it is required.

The social history entails a review of the patient's past and current activities, including smoking, alcohol and drug use, marital status, employment, living situation, and social supports. The clinician should describe the part of the social history that is clinically relevant. If it is not clinically relevant, bill at a lower level. Writing "social history is negative" is not a true statement or creditable as social history, as every patient has a social history.

I audited a note in which the social history read "He has a nice extended family that cares about him." At first glance, I wondered if there was any social history in that statement. However, as I read on in the note, I recognized that how the patient would be cared for after the discharge was relevant. The discussion of the patient's caring family was very much to the point and I counted it as social history.

Using a previous PFSH in an electronic health record is simple, but can result in tears if not done appropriately and correctly. Typically, the staff member opens a template when rooming the patient, then opens the past medical, family, and social history. "Any changes?" The note for the sore throat now has a page and a half of history that may not be relevant to today's problems. Remember, the Guidelines only allow using this history if the physician/provider reviews it with the patient. My rule of thumb: if you wouldn't have reviewed the past medical history before starting with an electronic health record, don't add it into the record for that day's visit. The Guidelines don't credit the clinician for copying the information from one visit to the next, but for reviewing it with the patient, and allow it to be used if that review is documented.

Interval History

Certain visits require only an interval history. For these visits, no past medical, family, or social history is required, as documented in the Documentation Guidelines and in the CPT® book. The HPI and ROS requirements for that level of history remain the same, but the PFSH is not required. When you look at the CPT® definition of certain codes, such as subsequent hospital visit, it describes, "an interval problem focused history" or "an interval detailed history" to meet the level of service requirements. The CPT® book does not define an interval history, but the Documentation Guidelines do define an interval history and list those codes for which an interval history is required:

> For certain categories of E/M services that include only an interval history, it is not necessary to record information about the PFSH. Those categories are subsequent hospital care, follow-up inpatient consultations and subsequent nursing facility care.

This makes sense. If the patient was admitted to the hospital in the last day or two and the physician documented the past medical, family, and social history, it would hardly be clinically relevant to re-document it the next day. (The Documentation Guidelines include subsequent consultation codes, but subsequent consultation codes were deleted in 2006. The Guidelines were written in 1995 and revised in 1997.)

How do we put these all together into a level of history? All histories need a chief complaint or a reason for the visit, explicitly stated or able to be inferred from the HPI. Remember, you need all components at or above the level for the history. The lowest level of the three—HPI, ROS, or PFSH—determines the level of history. Figure 3 summarizes the requirements for history.

FIGURE 3. Requirements for a Level of History

	History of Present Illness (HPI)	Review of Systems (ROS)	Past Medical, Family, and Social History (PFSH)
Problem Focused	1–3 elements	N/A	N/A
Expanded Problem Focused	1–3 elements	1 system	N/A
Detailed	4 elements or 3 chronic dx	2–9 systems	1 or 2
Comprehensive	4 elements or 3 chronic dx	At least 10 systems	2 or 3

Auditing the Exam

"Normal Exam Template"

Use caution when building and using EMR templates. Using the same exam for all patients suggests cloned notes. If a physician is using a normal template, it must be edited to reflect that day's exam. This is true for both inpatient and office notes. When using a paper template, use caution with check marks for "normal." Describe the exam for the body area in the presenting problem.

Significant differences exist in the exam portions of the 1995 and the 1997 Guidelines. The auditor is permitted, and your Medicare Contractor is required, to use whichever set of Guidelines is most beneficial to the provider.

1995 Exam

The 1995 exam confounds auditors by its lack of specificity. The entire description of the exam, including instructions, is barely one and one-half pages long. It divides the exam into body areas and organ systems as listed below. So far, so good, right?

For the purpose of examination as related to E/M coding, the following **organ systems** and **body areas** are recognized:

Organ Systems
1) Constitutional (e.g., vitals, general appearance)
2) Eyes
3) Ears, nose, mouth and throat
4) Cardiovascular
5) Respiratory
6) Gastrointestinal
7) Genitourinary
8) Musculoskeletal
9) Skin
10) Neurologic
11) Psychiatric
12) Hematologic/lymphatic/immunologic

Body Areas
1) Head, including the face
2) Neck
3) Chest, including breasts and axillae
4) Abdomen
5) Genitalia, groin, and buttocks
6) Back, including spine
7) Each extremity

The definition of a problem focused exam is easy. According to the 1995 Guidelines, it is a limited exam of the affected body area or organ system. We can see many examples of this when we audit. The patient returns to the office for a re-check, and the physician examines only a single organ system. Or, a patient presents with a problem that is minor or affects only one system, such as a contact dermatitis, and the physician examines only the skin.

The next two categories begin to cause problems. An expanded problem focused exam is defined as "a limited examination of the affected body area or organ system and other symptomatic or related organ system(s)." Notice, no specific number of body areas or organ systems is mentioned here. The Guidelines don't say how many body areas or organ systems you need to examine, only that it is a limited exam of the affected and related areas/systems.

Okay, how about the detailed exam? Is there any help there? The Guidelines say that a detailed exam is "an *extended* examination of the affected body area(s) and other symptomatic or related organ system(s)." Again, the Guidelines do not explicitly state how many or explain the difference between a **limited** exam for expanded problem focused and an **extended** exam for the detailed.

Some help can be found in the final definition of the comprehensive exam. A comprehensive exam is *a general multi-system exam or complete examination of a single organ system.* This definition gives us a few pieces of critical information. First, for a multi-system exam to be comprehensive, it must have 8 or more of the 12 organ systems examined, *not* body areas. The definition of a complete, single organ system exam is never defined with any more clarity or detail or description than above. This leaves auditors, physicians, non-physician practitioners, and contractors to make their own interpretations of what a complete examination of a single organ system is.

The comprehensive definition gives us some hints about how many areas/systems need to be examined for both the expanded problem focused and the detailed exams: two to seven. Some auditors and contractors have interpreted this to mean that an expanded problem focused exam is two to four body areas/organ systems and a detailed is five to seven body areas/organ systems examined. While this is a reasonable way to differentiate between the two levels of exam, it is not an official, CMS-sanctioned way of doing it. *Only use it if it is the system your contractor has adopted.* Some auditors make the determination on a note-by-note basis, allowing a detailed exam when, say, three areas/systems are examined but one of the areas seems to be an extended exam.

The auditor using the 1995 exam Guidelines frequently makes judgments and assumptions. Some practices have addressed this by developing internal, defensible policies about the difference between the expanded problem focused exam and the detailed exam. Internal, defensible, and documented consistency in this area could serve a practice well in a government audit.

Expanded Problem Focused vs. Detailed, 1995

This is one of the two areas auditors struggle with when using the 1995 Guidelines. As we saw in the above section, the difference between the two is a word: a *limited* exam of two to seven systems or an *extended* exam of two to seven systems. What should you do?

Option 1: If sanctioned by your contractor, use two to four organ systems or body areas examined for expanded problem focused (EPF) and five to seven organ systems or body areas for detailed. Count any single examined element documented as meeting the requirements for that area or system. For example, "vital signs" allows you to count the constitutional system. A description of the throat allows you to count the ENT system. Check your contractor's web site. Many of them post their audit sheets so you can see if your contractor uses this system. You can feel confident using this method *only* if your contractor does, too.

Option 2: Give credit for a detailed exam if a single organ system is detailed and one other system is examined. This is useful for specialists. What is detailed? Decide that for your practice, document your policy, and use it consistently. If you are a GYN office, a detailed exam could include four or more specific GYN elements, such as vagina, cervix, external genitalia, uterus, adnexa, bladder, or urethra, and one other organ system. If you are a Cardiac office, a detailed exam could include four or more specific Cardiac exam elements, such as palpation, auscultation, carotids, abdominal aorta, femoral pulses, pedal pulses, extremities, and one other system. Document your policy.

Option 3: A more conservative approach is to use the 1997 Guidelines for any notes for which there is a question about whether the exam is EPF or detailed. If the exam is comprehensive by the 1995 Guidelines, use that. If the exam is EPF, use that. But if you are in that gray area between EPF and comprehensive, go to the 1997 exam. This is a conservative, but defensible approach.

Can you set an internal policy? *In my opinion*, in the absence of more specifics from your contractor or CMS, it is your safest course. It gives you internal consistency and validity. Develop a reasonable, clinically sound, defensible policy with input and approval from your medical director; write it down; communicate it to physicians; and give it to your auditors. It will speed up their auditing because they won't have to sit and decide each time, "Is it detailed?" It will increase your internal consistency because all of your auditors will have audited these exams in the same way.

Comprehensive Exams, 1995

There is no guidance about what constitutes a "complete examination of a single organ system." If you are in a specialty practice and using the 1995 Guidelines, I suggest you use the 1997 Guidelines instead. This would be the most conservative, safest course. Rather than developing your own policy about single specialty exams, educate your providers about what they need to meet the single specialty exam requirements in the 1997 Guidelines.

If you are using the 1995 Guidelines and want to meet the requirements for a multi-system exam, you need to have eight organ systems (not body areas) documented. There is no guidance about the amount of detail that needs to be documented in each system. A single element in the organ system examined counts for the entire system. For example, "Lungs–clear" counts as respiratory. There is no CMS explanation about what exam constitutes the organ system for GI an what exam is the body area abdominal, for example. I often find that using the 1995 Guidelines and the multi-system exam when auditing high-level services is the most beneficial for providers. When auditing admissions or Level 4 or Level 5 consults, or new patient visits, this strategy frequently results in the highest level of service.

Exam Labels

Sometimes a physician will label an exam element in a different system than I typically audit it. A physician may dictate, "Neurological: Alert and oriented times three." I usually credit the psychiatric system for orientation and mood. I ignore the physician labels and give credit for the exam elements in a consistent fashion from note to note. I use the placement of exam elements in the 1997 Guidelines as my guide as to which organ system to credit. This provides a consistent, defensible method for assigning exam elements to an organ system/body area when using the 1995 Guidelines.

Organ Systems and Body Areas

Auditors understand clearly that they cannot count body areas to meet the comprehensive exam; but, how do they decide if an exam description is an organ system or body area? Here's *my opinion and policy on how to do that.* My system is to start by crediting organ systems. I use the body areas if the description doesn't fit in any organ system. For example, "Neck—supple" or "Head—atraumatic" would both be credited as body areas because there is no organ system to describe them. However, for "Neck—no lymph nodes palpable," I would credit lymph in the organ system rather than neck. Here are other examples of what I do *in my own internal policy:*

For: "Neck—carotids"   I credit cardiovascular.
For: "Extremities—no edema"   I credit cardiovascular.
For: "GI: no tenderness, HSM,   I credit GI as an organ system.
normal bowel sounds"

No one at CMS or any contractor has confirmed this—it is *my policy.* This is what I do:
- Give credit for the organ system first.
- Use a description of an element once.
- Use the 1997 Guidelines to decide in what system to credit an exam description.
- Use these policies consistently from note to note.

It is clear why the exam component of the 1995 Guidelines is giving auditors gray hair all around the country!

Now that we have cleared up all of the ambiguity in the 1995 Guidelines, what does the provider need to document in the exam? The provider must describe specific abnormalities and describe negative body areas/organ systems related to the affected area/system. It is not acceptable to simply say "Lungs—abnormal." The provider must document how the lungs sound. For those body areas/organ systems that are unrelated to the presenting problem or affected system, a simple notation of "normal" is acceptable.

1997 Exam

The 1997 Guidelines brought providers and auditors specificity. By my informal polling, auditors prefer the 1997 Guidelines because they removed the ambiguity of the 1995 exam elements, and physicians and other providers liked them less because they felt that the newer Guidelines reduced their work to "counting bullets."

The multi-system exam did remove the doubt between the problem focused and the expanded problem focused exam and the detailed exam. It is easy to audit an exam with the 1997 Guidelines and know for sure if the provider met the criteria for each level. For the multi-system exam, 1–5 elements identified by a bullet must be performed; for expanded problem focused, 6–11 elements; for detailed, 12–17 elements; and for comprehensive, document two bullets in nine systems.

The 1997 Guidelines also included single specialty exams. These exams did not prove to be as useful as some specialists had hoped, particularly for the comprehensive exam. The instructions for reaching the comprehensive exam are difficult to explain to physicians and NPPs. Here's an example: *Perform all elements identified by a bullet; document every element in each box with a shaded border and at least one element in each box with an unshaded border.*

The instructions for each organ system (how many, etc.) are listed after the organ system is described. For many specialists, the amount of detail required for the comprehensive level exam was harder to do and document than the 1995 multi-system exam. This is not uniformly true: the eye exam, psychiatry exam, ENT exam, and some others are useful to specialists in documenting the relevant clinical work. Physicians, NPPs, and auditors should look carefully at these single specialty exams to determine their potential benefit to the provider.

Any single specialty exam can be used by any provider of any specialty. That is, the cardiac exam is not limited for use by cardiologists. The provider does not have to label the exam—the auditor can determine which exam was used. Look carefully at the single specialty exam requirements, particularly for the comprehensive exam. They require all bullets in certain categories, all performed in other categories, and at least one documented in these.

Normal, Negative Exam Descriptions

Exam Guidelines outlined in the 1995 version are relevant to the 1997 exam Guidelines. Positives and negatives related to the presenting problem or affected area/system must be explicitly described and negative findings unrelated to the presenting problem or affected body area/system can be indicated as "normal" or "negative."

FIGURE 4. Comparison of 1995 and 1997 Exam Guidelines

Type of Examination	1995 Description of Examination	1995 Guidelines	1997 Guidelines
Problem Focused	Limited exam of affected body area or organ system	1 body area or organ system	1–5 bullets
Expanded Problem Focused	Limited exam of affected body area or organ system and other symptomatic or related organ systems	2–7 body areas or organ systems	6 bullets
Detailed	Extended exam of affected body area(s) and other symptomatic or related organ systems	2–7 body areas or organ systems	6 areas w/2 bullets **or** 12 in 2 systems
Comprehensive	General multi-system exam or complete exam of a single organ system	8 organ systems	9 areas w/2 bullets each

Medical Decision Making

According to the Documentation Guidelines, the medical decision making component of an E/M code refers to

The complexity of establishing a diagnosis and/or selecting a management option as measured by:
* *The number of possible diagnoses and/or the number of management options that must be considered;*

- *The amount and/or complexity of medical records, diagnostic tests, and/or other information that must be obtained, reviewed and analyzed; and*
- *The risk of significant complications, morbidity and/or mortality, as well as comorbidities, associated with the patient's presenting problem(s), the diagnostic procedure(s) and/or the possible management options.*

There are four levels of medical decision making (MDM), each requiring two of the three elements of medical decision making:

- Straightforward
- Low complexity
- Moderate complexity
- High complexity

The first of the three components in establishing medical decision making is the number of diagnoses or management options considered during the visit. The Guidelines assume that new problems to the examining physician (not to the patient) are more complex than established problems, that undiagnosed problems are more complex than known ones, and that problems that are worsening or failing to improve are more complex than improving problems. The Guidelines state that the status of the patient's problems should be documented for established problems, such as improved, worsening, etc. Management options should also be documented, such as referrals to consultants and any instructions, therapies, or medications ordered.

How does an auditor know if the problem is new or established to the examining provider? Sometimes it takes a crystal ball! If the patient is new to the provider, it is safe to assume that the problem is new to the examining provider. In some notes, the HPI makes it clear, because the problem is described as a new onset. Or, the provider states that he has never seen the patient for this problem. There are sometimes clues in the assessment. "This longstanding problem . . ." or "This exacerbation of. . . ." Both of those phrases would indicate the patient's problem was longstanding, and you may be able to assume that this provider has treated the patient for the problem previously. If I cannot tell definitively, I err on the side of caution and assume that the problem is established to the provider.

Some problems by their very nature are new and acute, sudden-onset problems. The HPI makes this clear: "The patient awoke with chest pain and reports that he has never experienced pain like this before."

What about recurrences, such as recurrent urinary tract infections? If a patient has a history of recurrent UTIs (and the examiner has treated the problem before) but the patient's symptoms resolved with treatment, I count a recurrence as a new problem. However, for chronic problems with ongoing symptoms, an exacerbation is an established, worsening problem. This is another judgment. CMS does not provide that level of detail in its guidance.

Whether a patient problem "needs work up," which is a higher level of medical decision making, depends on whether a work up is planned for after the day's visit. When I audit, I do not count diagnostic tests completed at the visit as "with work up planned." Some Emergency Department auditors may credit the work up done in the ED but there is no official citation allowing or disallowing that.

The second element in determining MDM is the amount and/or complexity of data to be reviewed during the encounter. The popular point system we see in many audit sheets is not part of the original 1995 or 1997 Guidelines, but was developed by a private organization as a way of quantifying the amount of data ordered or reviewed. This point system has been widely adopted by auditors and some contractors, but has no basis in the Guidelines themselves.

Ordering or reviewing a lab test, x-ray, or test from the medicine section of the CPT® book is an indication of complexity. The review of these tests may be indicated by an explicit statement, e.g., "glucose today 110," or by initialing and dating the report with the test results.

Obtaining and reviewing old records increases the amount of data that must be reviewed, as does the decision to discuss test results findings with a testing physician or personally reviewing a tracing, image, or slide that was or will be interpreted by someone else. The Guidelines state specifically, however, that simply stating "Old records reviewed" is insufficient detail without a description of the information obtained. Discussions with caregivers and family, similarly, can also increase the complexity level of the data component if there is a description of the relevant clinical information obtained from the family member.

If a clinician has independently reviewed an image, tracing, or specimen interpreted by another clinician, the point system assigns two points for that clinician. This might occur when a patient presents to a neurologist and brings her MRI images for review. A radiologist has previously interpreted the image, and the neurologist may not bill for a professional interpretation. But, by noting that the images—not simply the report—were reviewed, the complexity increases. An internist may admit a patient and review a chest x-ray that a radiologist will interpret later. If the clinician is billing for the service, such as an EKG in the office, most auditors give one point, not two. This is not in the Guidelines, but is an interpretation of the Guidelines.

Remember that not all contractors use the point system. The Guidelines use these words to describe the amount of data reviewed: minimal or none, limited, moderate, and extensive. The point system is used to quantify those words.

The final element of MDM is the risk of complications and/ or morbidity or mortality. This section, like so many sections of the Guidelines, is divided into three parts: 1) the risks related to the presenting problem(s); 2) the risks related to diagnostic procedures ordered; and 3) the risks related to the management options selected. This table of risk is included on the audit sheet.

Some new auditors think they need an item from all three columns in the table of risk, but that's not necessary. As you read the note, the level of risk is determined from all parts of the note. Notice the category descriptions: the presenting problem, the diagnostic tests ordered, and the treatment planned. The presenting problem is most related to the history. For example, the patient presents with a chronic illness or an undiagnosed new problem. You will find the status of the chronic illness or problem in either the history or in the assessment. The diagnostic tests and treatment ordered are usually found in the plan. Circle one or more descriptions from the table of risk and use the description in the row with the highest risk.

Each of these three types of risk has four levels: 1) minimal, 2) low, 3) moderate, and 4) high. These are not to be confused with the final MDM determinations of low, straightforward, moderate, and high. To determine the level of risk of "significant complications, morbidity, and/ or mortality," find the highest level of presenting problem, diagnostic test, or management option that describes the patient encounter you are auditing. Select the highest one—you need only one. The table of risk is included in the 1997 Documentation Guidelines and on the audit sheet.

When it comes time to select the medical decision making, use a grid on your audit sheet. In each column, mark the level of diagnoses or treatment options, the amount of complexity, and the risk of complications with a circle. If you have two or three circles at the same level, select that level of risk (low, straightforward, moderate, high). If the three circles are all at different levels, select the level of risk in which the middle circle is located.

FIGURE 5. Determination of Medical Decision Making

Type of Decision Making	Number of Diagnoses or Management Options	Amount and/or Complexity of Data to Be Reviewed	Risk of Complications and/or Morbidity/ Mortality
Straightforward/Minimal	Minimal	Minimal or None	Minimal
Low Complexity	Limited	Limited	Low
Moderate Complexity	Multiple	Moderate	Moderate
High Complexity	Extensive	Extensive	High

What about prescription drug management? Prescription drug management appears in the table of risk under treatment options as moderate MDM. There is no discussion of whether it is a new prescription or a refill, or about the type of prescription drug. Some payers or auditors don't want to credit all prescriptions, only new prescriptions or prescriptions for a "serious" problem. There is no basis on the Guidelines themselves for this. The Guidelines count prescription drug management under the table of risk as moderate MDM, and so do I.

Does MDM Need to Be One of the Three Key Components?

Some visits require only two of the three key components, such as established patient visits and subsequent hospital care. Some groups have an internal policy that MDM must be one of the key components, and in support of this, use CMS's statement that medical necessity is the overarching criterion for selecting a level of E/M service. However, medical necessity is not synonymous with medical decision making. The medical necessity for performing the key components of history and exam are determined by the nature of the presenting problem, the patient's own personal history, and the clinical judgment of the provider. The medical decision making—that is the diagnostics ordered, the assessment, and the plan—are formulated as a **result** of the nature of the presenting problem, the patient's past medical history, and the history and exam performed at that visit. MDM is the outcome of the visit and is not a substitute for medical necessity. If CMS had wanted medical decision making to be a substitute, the *Medicare Claims Processing Manual* would read, "medical decision making is the overarching criterion in selecting an E/M service" instead of medical necessity. If CMS had wanted medical decision making to be a substitute for medical necessity, either medical decision making would be **required** in determining the code or all codes would require all three components.

Physicians do need to use their electronic health records in a way that more clearly documents what happened at the visit. In most cases that means documenting what would have been dictated and being prudent in copying and clicking. Length of note doesn't win a prize. Coders need to recognize the difference between the medical necessity of performing a history and exam based on the nature of the presenting problem and the patient's condition and medical decision making that is the clinical outcome of the encounter. Organizations should seriously consider how policies and incentives are affecting coding for E/M services.

The Use and Abuses of Templates

No sooner were the Guidelines published than the first template rolled off the assembly line of a word processor. Coding consultants and educators got busy. "Doctor, just fill out this form, and all of your visits can be a level four!" Some physician notes began to take on a predictability that was almost scary! It was inevitable that the OIG would put this on their Work Plan.

The *Medicare Claims Processing Manual* carries this instruction about selecting a level of service:

> *Medical necessity of a service is the overarching criterion for payment in addition to the individual requirements of a CPT® code. It would not be medically necessary or appro-priate to bill a higher level of evaluation and management service when a lower level of service is warranted. The volume of documentation should not be the primary influence upon which a specific level of service is billed. Documentation should support the level of service reported. The service should be documented during, or as soon as practicable after it is provided in order to maintain an accurate medical record.*

CMS does not expect physicians to bill a higher level of service when a lower level of service is all that is required based on the patient's presenting problem and the nature of the patient's underlying illnesses. This can be a problem for new patient visits when practices have patients complete a health history form. Using the form for the history, and following an exam template, many new patients and consults can be documented at a Level 4. However, Medicare wants the provider to consider whether it was medically necessary to take that level of history and exam for each patient. If a patient has a minor presenting problem, it would not be necessary or typical for the provider to take and document a high level of history and exam.

Established patients require only two of the three key components. That means that a provider can select a code based on any two of three components. However, it would not be medically necessary to document all detailed or comprehensive histories and exams in order to meet the requirements of 99214 or 99215. The encounter documentation should show the necessity for that level of service.

Some paper templates use so many check-off boxes that the patient's condition is not clearly described. Be sure to document an adequate history of the present illness and describe the problem and the status of the problems in the assessment. These forms will often allow physicians to think they can bill a Level 4 visit. Be sure there is adequate written documentation to support a Level 4 visit.

Some physicians use a "macro" in their word processing program for their review of systems. They will dictate the HPI and then say, "Normal female ROS." There are two potential problems with this: 1) Does the provider ask all of the questions each time? and 2) Do any of the "normal systems" contradict the HPI elements? I see this problem in notes documented with an electronic medical record. The HPI will say, "Patient has 3-day history of abdominal pain, constipation, and gas." The GI section of the ROS will contradict this, "GI—no diarrhea, constipation, pain, nausea, vomiting, etc." If the HPI and the ROS contradict each other, and I can see from the physician notes that a template is used, I will not give credit for any of the items.

Using an electronic medical record allows providers to "click" on fields and include those aspects in the note, such as the patient's past medical, family, and social history. The provider need only click on a button that indicates, "Reviewed, no changes needed" and the entire past medical, family, and social history entered at a previous visit becomes part of that day's note. The PFSH may have been entered by that provider or another provider in a shared medical record. I ask physicians two questions when I see this: 1) Was it necessary for today's visit to review the past medical, family, and social history? and 2) Did you review it, specifically?

The same problem exists in some electronic medical records for the exam. I recently reviewed a series of 10 notes documented using an EMR. For all 10, the provider had indicated that all of the psychiatry elements were examined. "Normal judgment and insight, intact

memory, alert and oriented to time place and person, normal mood."
The presenting problems were varied: elbow pain, URIs. One of the
patients, for whom a normal psychiatric exam was documented, was two
years old! I wonder how the provider tested the two-year-old's memory
and orientation! And why? For those types of notes, I tend to ignore
the elements that do not seem relevant. I strongly recommend that the
provider document only those elements that would seem reasonable
and necessary to another provider.

Using Time as the Determining Factor

Providers can use time in selecting some E/M codes when certain
conditions are met. More than half of the visit must be spent in
counseling and coordination of care. The provider must document
the total time of the visit, the fact that more than 50% of the visit was
spent in counseling, and the nature of the discussion. Remember, for
Medicare, the beneficiary must be present.

The CPT® book defines this counseling in this way:

Discussion with patient and/or family regarding:
- Diagnosis results, impressions, recommended diagnostic studies
- Prognosis
- Risks and benefits of management
- Instructions for management
- Importance of compliance
- Risk factor reduction
- Patient and family education

Time is not a factor in ED services. For the other E/M services, the
typical time for the visit is listed in the CPT® book. If you use time to
select a code, use those times.

What are some examples of visits that might qualify as visits in
which time is the determining factor?
- A patient is seen with a new onset problem, sent for diagnostic
  tests, and asked to return to the office when the test results are
  available. At the first visit, the physician takes the patient's history,
  examines the patient, and orders the tests. At the return visit,
  the physician does not re-take the history and may perform only
  a focused exam. The second visit is mostly discussion with the
  patient about the diagnosis and optimal treatment. The second
  visit can be coded using time as the determining factor.

- A patient returns to an Oncologist office after an initial diagnosis. The majority of the visit is spent discussing treatment options: surgery, radiation, chemotherapy, or some combination. The physician reviews the risks and benefits of each treatment and answers the patient's questions. This visit can be coded using time.
- A patient with several chronic illnesses, including hypertension, diabetes, and high cholesterol, comes in for a regular follow up. The patient's illnesses are not in good control. The physician spends most of the visit discussing the importance of complying with the treatment regimen and the risks of failure to comply.

Using time as the determining factor trumps the three key components.
What do you need to document?
- Total time for the visit.
- Statement that more than 50% of the visit was counseling.
- Description of the nature of the counseling.

Here are some samples of appropriate dictation:
"I spent 20 minutes face-to-face with the patient, over half of which was counseling/coordination of care."
"I spent 15 minutes with the patient, over half discussing her diagnosis and treatment."
"I spent 30 minutes with the patient and family, over half of which was discussing whether surgery was a good option at this time."
"We spent more than 50% of our 40-minute visit discussing the prognosis, plan, additional treatment, and the overall outlook for Stage IV non-small cell lung cancer."

These documentation examples *fail to satisfy* the requirement to use time as the determining factor:
"I spent 20 minutes in supportive counseling."
"Had a lengthy discussion with the patient."
"I spent 15 minutes talking about the treatment options." (How long was the total time?)

Determining Time

For office visit and outpatient consultations, the time that matters is **face-to-face** time in the exam room.

For hospital services, **unit time** is the time that matters. This includes time at the bedside, reviewing the chart, and communicating with other professionals and family. In the hospital, time does not include being in other departments, such as Radiology or lab. CMS requires that over half of the unit time is spent in face-to-face discussions.

To review, you must document the total time in the chart and state that the visit was for counseling and coordination of care. You must state that over 50% of the visit was spent in counseling. You must describe the nature of the discussion you had with the patient. No history or examination elements are required.

Look at Prior Visits

Most auditors now review a prior visit when auditing an E/M note, to check for copying and pasting that is excessive. This should be a regular feature of your compliance plan. I heard a speaker describing their audit process. For each section of the note, HPI, ROS, PFSH, exam, assessment and plan, the auditor reviews the previous note and assesses the section as: unique, identical or similar. Except for PFSH, identical is not credited. For entries that are similar, the auditor uses judgment to decide whether to credit the information.

Final Word to Auditors

Auditors have a heavy responsibility for both revenue and compliance. Sometimes we let it get into our heads and weigh us down. Sometimes we let it go to our heads and feel pretty darn self-important!

I think the best auditors are pro-doctor, which is not the same as pro-revenue. Our job is to educate and inform our providers, help them earn deserved revenue, and keep them out of trouble. I try to keep a positive, respectful attitude and never think that I know more than the provider.

The Guidelines have so many gray areas that it has turned my hair gray. (I've stopped blaming my kids, and now blame the Guidelines.) Here is my advice on how to deal with gray areas:

- Attend an auditing seminar every two or three years. It is amazing to me how much more I learned at subsequent sessions.
- Read and re-read the Documentation Guidelines themselves. They are the source documents. They answer many questions that coders, auditors and providers have.
- Check your contractor's web site. If it posts an audit tool, use its tool or a standard tool. Do not make up your own tool—the Guidelines are too detailed.
- Use an audit tool every time. Let me say that again. Use an audit tool for each and every note that you audit.

- Develop written policies for gray areas.
- Don't make it harder on physicians than the Guidelines already do.
- Don't develop a negative attitude.
- Have a second auditor re-audit a certain percentage of your notes. I always find that useful and educational.
- Cultivate a physician partner.

WHY THE OIG CARES

In a recent Office of Inspector General (OIG) report on trends in E/M coding, the OIG noted that payment for E/M services in 2010 was $33.5 billion and that E/M services were vulnerable to abuse. Paying providers for the service provided and documented is central to the OIG's mission. When it comes to E/M services, the definition for each level of service is complex and subject to error. And yet, by volume and by revenue, the E/M services comprise a large portion of the monies spent by the Medicare program. At one CMS Open Door Forum, a CMS official stated that E/M services account for 30% of all physician payments.

Medicare wants to pay physicians for the level of service provided and documented and uses the Documentation Guidelines as a way to verify the validity of coding these services. The CMS manual also reminds providers that medical necessity is the linchpin for selecting an E/M code. Here's what the manual states:

> *Medical necessity of a service is the overarching criterion for payment in addition to the individual requirements of a CPT® code. It would not be medically necessary or appro-priate to bill a higher level of evaluation and management service when a lower level of service is warranted. The volume of documentation should not be the primary influence upon which a specific level of service is billed. Documentation should support the level of service reported. The service should be documented during, or as soon as practicable after it is provided in order to maintain an accurate medical record.*

Providers should use medical necessity as the first criterion in selecting a code, and then ensure that their documentation meets the criteria for the level of service provided and billed.

Medical necessity is not the same as medical decision making. Medical necessity is shown in the HPI, the assessment, the plan, and the nature of the presenting problem. Medical decision making is one of the three key components, with a specific set of elements.

RED FLAGS

In auditing E/M services, these are the kinds of problems that raise a red flag:

- Handwritten notes that are difficult to read.
- Limited history of the present illness in a note generated using an electronic medical record (EMR).
- Ancillary staff recording the HPI and limited physician/ NPP-generated HPI.
- A templated ROS that contradicts information listed in the HPI.
- Most of the history documented with "check-off" boxes.
- High level of documentation for minor presenting problems.
- Notes that all seem the same.
- Exam elements documented using EMR that are unrelated to the presenting problem, such as, "Normal external ears/nose" when the presenting problem is unrelated to the ENT system.
- Assessments that list all of the patient's medical problems, not just problems addressed at the current visit.
- Assessments that do not indicate if the patient's problems are better, worsening, etc.
- Treatment plans that are not explicit.
- Assessments that say only "Stable. Continue current plans."
- Two notes on the same patient from different dates of service are similar. Or identical.

COMPLIANCE RESPONSE

Educate

There is no substitute for education when it comes to the Documentation Guidelines. Physicians and NPPs must take the time to learn these Guidelines. They were developed in 1995 and 1997, and yet there are still physicians and NPPs who are unclear about the documentation required for the codes they use most often. I met with a physician whose contractor had requested pre-payment note for 99244 visits. When I reviewed the notes, they audited as 99243s. He asked me, "Could I have been expected to know these rules?"

The most effective education takes place after hours, off-site, and is sufficient in length to present the entire system and answer questions. Typically, one and one-half to three hours work well. Groups of 10 to 30 providers are the best. Groups encourage questions, inform all providers by the questions of some providers, and allow everyone to hear the same answer to all questions, re-question, and clarify. "What if" questions work well in these classes, e.g., "What if I'm called back to the hospital in the evening?" "What if the patient is emotional and the visit takes a lot longer than is normal?" or "What if I do a procedure on the same day as an office visit?"

Re-Audit

Organizations usually have a policy that defines what percentage of errors trigger a re-audit. Some groups differentiate between compliance errors (services billed at a higher level than documented or in a wrong category—overcoding) and revenue errors (services billed at a lower level than documented—undercoding). Let compliance errors of more than 10% to 20% trigger a re-audit. It is most useful to re-audit in the selected area of the error. That is, many physicians understand the Documentation Guidelines for new and established patient visits. Hospital services may have more errors. Re-audit those services that have errors rather than services that are understood and billed correctly. It is another way to use your limited compliance resources wisely.

Give Individual Feedback

Educate in a group, but give individual feedback on specific notes one-on-one. The auditor should bring a copy of the note, the audit sheet, and a copy of the Documentation Guidelines to the meeting with the provider. The auditor should tell the provider specifically what components of the note failed to meet the level of service the provider selected, and what additional components are needed for that level of service. Repeat this sequence of audits and feedback as often as needed.

Address Persistent Errors

If a provider remains persistent with level of service or category errors, audit all of this person's claims before submission. Review the chapter on the OIG Work Plan and your compliance plan for suggestions about sanctions and governance for physicians who have repeated coding and billing errors.

> *See Appendix 1,*
> *E/M Documentation Auditing Worksheet*

CHAPTER 4

New Patient Visits

The question seems simple enough: Is the patient a new or an established patient? Should the patient be charged using the new patient codes, 99201–99205, or the established patient codes, 99211–99215? But there are pervasive misconceptions about whether a patient is new or established. To complicate matters, the CPT® and Medicare definitions are different, with payers following the Medicare definition in processing claims.

Here's the citation from the CPT® book:

Solely for the purposes of distinguishing between new and established patients, professional services are those face-to-face services rendered by physicians and other qualified health care professionals who may evaluation and management services reported by a specific CPT code(s). and reported by a specific CPT® code(s). A new patient is one who has never received any professional services from the physician/qualified health care professional or another physician/qualified healthcare professional of the exact same specialty and subspecialty who belongs to the same group practice, within the past three years.

A professional service is defined as a face-to-face service provided by a physician or non-physician practitioner (NPP) and billed with a CPT® code. This *does not include* reading an EKG, interpreting an x-ray, or any other non face-to-face diagnostic test. It *does* include services provided in an Emergency Department (ED), hospital visits, surgical services, consults, office visits, and any other face-to-face service provided and billed using a CPT® code.

Medicare's definition does not differentiate subspecialty.

A Definition of New Patient for Selection of E/M Visit Code

Interpret the phrase "new patient" to mean a patient who has not received any professional services, i.e., E/M service or other face-to-face service (e.g., surgical procedure) from the physician or physician group practice (same physician specialty) within the previous 3 years. For example, if a professional component of a previous procedure is billed in a 3 year time period, e.g., a lab interpretation is billed and no E/M service or other face-to-face service with the patient is performed, then this patient remains a new patient for the initial visit. An interpretation of a diagnostic test, reading an x-ray or EKG etc., in the absence of an E/M service or other face-to-face service with the patient does not affect the designation of a new patient.

Within a group practice, the definition distinguishes between the specialties of the physicians providing the service. All physicians/practitioners enrolled in the Medicare program are enrolled with a two-digit specialty designation. It's important that these are accurate during the Medicare enrollment process, because the specialty designation affects claims processing and reimbursement. Although the CPT definition uses the terms "exact same specialty or subspecialty," only specialties recognized by Medicare as distinct specialties, based on the two-digit taxonomy code, are used.

Patients who were seen first in the hospital and later in the office are defined as established patients at the time of the office visit. For example, a patient who has never been seen by any physician in your practice is admitted to the hospital by an internist, Dr. Abbott, over the weekend. Upon discharge, the patient is instructed to follow up with the practice the following week. When Dr. Abbott or any of Dr. Abbott's Internal Medicine partners sees the patient for the first time in the office, the patient is considered an established patient because of that prior hospital visit by Dr. Abbott.

A Cardiologist performs a consult on a hospitalized patient. The patient is discharged and goes to the Cardiology office for follow up. That patient visit is an established patient visit.

A Family Practitioner (FP) leaves a solo practice and joins an existing Family Practice group in the same town. Many of the FP's patients transfer care to the new practice to see their old physician. They are established patients to the new practice when they see their old physician for their first visit in the new practice. Why? They have received a professional service from this physician in the past three years. The fact that the group changed for billing purposes does not change the definition of a new patient. The new tax ID does not make a difference in this case.

Here are examples of new patients:

A patient returns to the practice after a three-year, one-month absence.

A patient in a multi-specialty group is typically seen by an Internal Medicine doctor. He self-refers to a GI doctor. He is a new patient to the GI doctor, because the GI doctor is a different specialty in the same group. And remember, self-referrals are not consults.

A multi-specialty group includes Pediatricians, Internists, and OB/GYN doctors. When patients who are seen by the Pediatrician turn 18, they are typically transferred to another doctor of a different specialty. The first visit to the Internist or OB/GYN doctor is a new patient visit. The patient may be a long-established patient to the practice, but when seen by a physician of a different specialty, a new patient visit can be billed. Some groups bill this as an established patient visit for public relations reasons, but from a coding perspective it is a new patient.

A physician reads EKGs on contract with the local hospital. He reads the EKG of a patient who later makes an appointment to see that physician. Reading an EKG does not constitute a face-to-face service, so the physician may bill a new patient visit for that initial encounter.

Another common myth about new patients is that if the patient presents for a new problem, a physician may bill a new patient visit. This is incorrect. The differentiation of a new or established problem is not a factor in determining if a patient is new or established.

A Primary Care group that starts a Walk-in Clinic or Urgent Care Center will realize that from the specialty perspective, there is no designation of Urgent Care for the physician. Most of the physicians working in an Urgent Care center are Internists, FPs or Pediatricians.

WHY DOES THE OIG CARE?

The reimbursement for new patient visits is higher than for established patient visits. Figure 1 shows a comparison of relative value units (RVUs) for new and established patients.

These RVUs and national payment rates are the most recent as the book is prepared for press. To look up the latest RVUs and payment rates, go to http://www.cms.gov/apps/physician-fee-schedule/search/search-criteria.aspx

Whenever there is a financial advantage to the practice if the billing is done incorrectly, the Office of Inspector General (OIG) and your carrier are interested in you billing it correctly! In addition to following the new patient definition in the CPT® book, the *CMS Internet-Only Manual* also adds this guidance for physicians in group practices:

30.6.5 Physicians in Group Practice
(Rev. 1, 10-01-03) Physicians in the same group practice who are in the same specialty must bill and be paid as though they were a single

FIGURE 1. New and Established Patient RVUs and Payment

COMPARISON OF NEW PATIENT VS. OLD PATIENT RVUS/PAYMENT		
CPT code	RVUs	National Payment
New Patients		
99201	1.23	43.98
99202	2.1	75.08
99203	3.05	109.05
99204	4.64	165.9
99205	5.83	208.45
Established Patients		
99211	0.56	20.02
99212	1.23	43.98
99213	2.04	72.94
99214	3.03	108.34
99215	4.09	146.24
All rates are national, non-facility rates for participating physicians.		

physician. If more than one evaluation and management (face-to-face) service is provided on the same day to the same patient by the same physician or more than one physician in the same specialty in the same group, only one evaluation and management service may be reported unless the evaluation and management services are for unrelated problems. Instead of billing separately, the physicians should select a level of service representative of the combined visits and submit the appropriate code for that level. Physicians in the same group practice but who are in different specialties may bill and be paid without regard to their membership in the same group.

If the CPT® definition of a new patient wasn't clear enough, the first sentence from this citation confirms that the government expects group physicians of the same specialty in the same practice to bill and be paid as if they were one physician.

RED FLAGS

Auditing new patient visits is the best way to know if your practice has a problem with them. But you can also ask two simple questions to see if you have a problem with new patient visits.

1. **Ask your physicians:** "If you see a patient over the weekend in the hospital for the first time, when you follow up in the office, is it a new or established patient?" If anyone says "new," you've got a problem.

2. **Ask your biller/data entry clerk/coder:** "Do we ever bill Medicare or a commercial insurer for a new patient and receive the paid claim as an established patient visit?" If the answer is yes, it's time for a review.

Factors that may cause variations in your practice data include:

- How long your providers have been in practice.
- Whether they are accepting new patients.
- Whether the practice typically sees new patients as consults rather than new patients.

Groups with multiple sites but a single group billing number are more likely to be unsure if the patient is new or established than groups in a single location. If your group has more than one location of same-specialty providers, it is important to look at this issue. Using an integrated EMR or practice management system is a useful step in addressing this. Similarly, if you employ many fill-in providers, perhaps at a Walk-In or Urgent Care Center, the physician selecting the code may not have access to the data about whether the patient was seen by someone of the same specialty in the past three years.

Some practices use the absence of an "old record" as proof that the patient has not been seen in the office in the past three years. This is not an effective or accurate measure. Paper medical records are subject to loss or misfiling. It is prudent to check the patient's financial account, as well.

COMPLIANCE RESPONSE

Most practices find that education of providers and billing staff solves the problem of whether a patient is new or established. It is critical for everyone to understand that "new patient" is not defined by making up a new chart or a new problem.

If your audit shows that you have billed new patient visits instead of established patient visits, consult a healthcare attorney. Consider implementing a check-off system for new patients based on the sample audit sheet at the end of this chapter. Ask the physician or non-physician practitioner to answer the questions on the audit sheet before selecting a new patient visit code for a short while. It will take only a few times filling out the audit sheet to reinforce the learning and definition of a new patient.

If you find, however, that you are billing established patients when the patient met the criteria for a new patient visit, count yourself lucky! You've found a source of revenue for the practice! Research the reasons for the incorrect billing. If it is a lack of knowledge of the rules, education is your solution. If the problem lies in multiple sites and providers who do not always know if the patient had been seen by a physician of the same specialty, solve that problem using your information system.

Whoever is posting the charge should be able to look up the patient's procedure and financial history and determine if the patient is new or established based on the rules. Keep in mind that the documentation requirements for new and established patients are different and you cannot simply charge a Level 3 new patient visit if a Level 3 established patient visit was charged.

So, what do you do if you find that you are routinely billing established patient visits when the patient met the criteria for a new patient?

You cannot simply assign a new code without looking at the documentation. And if you must audit every one of these notes, the cost will hardly justify the additional reimbursement. Consider an encounter form in which the provider circles not simply the procedure code, but the level of history, exam, and medical decision making performed.

For example, say a provider bills a patient for an established visit. The provider circles a detailed history, expanded problem-focused exam, and moderate medical decision making. This meets the qualification of a **99214**. If it turns out that the patient is new, the biller can assign the new patient code **99202**. If the provider circles detailed history, detailed exam, and moderate medical decision making, **99214**, and the patient is new, the biller can assign code **99203**. The reason for the difference is that new patients required that *all three key components* meet or exceed the guidelines, and established patients require only two of three key components be met.

COMPLIANCE PLAN AUDIT SHEET

Auditor Name:	Date of Audit:
Organization Name:	

New Patient Visit
To perform this audit, you will need: • The medical record for each visit • Access to the patient account • Old patient record, if the physician has joined your practice from another group Select 10 patients billed as new patients, and 10 billed as established patients. Complete this form for each patient.

Patient ID:	Provider ID:
Auditor ID:	Date of Audit:

Answer yes or no to the following questions by checking the appropriate box/circle:

From the medical record:		
Is there documentation of a previous, <u>face-to-face</u> professional service provided by <u>physician or non-physician practitioner</u> or <u>same-specialty physician or non-physician practitioner from the same group</u> in the past <u>three years</u>? Include all professional services, all locations for which a face-to-face service was provided, billed with a CPT® code. Do not include interpreting diagnostic tests, such as reading EKGs, interpreting x-rays, or providing an interpretation of a lab test.	❏ Yes	◯ No
From the patient account:		
Was the patient billed for a <u>face-to-face</u> professional service provided by <u>physician or non-physician practitioner</u> or <u>same-specialty physician or non-physician practitioner from the same group</u> in the past <u>three years</u>? Include all professional services, all locations for which a face-to-face service was provided, billed with a CPT® code. Do not include interpreting diagnostic tests, such as reading EKGs, interpreting x-rays, or providing an interpretation of a lab test.	❏ Yes	◯ No

<u>*Scoring Key*</u>
If you answered NO to both questions, bill a new patient visit.
If you answered YES to ONE question, bill an established patient visit.

CHAPTER 5

Consultations

According to the CPT book, "A consultation is a type of evaluation and management service provided at the request of another physician or appropriate source to either recommend care for a specific condition or problem or to determine whether to accept responsibility for ongoing management of the patient's entire care or for the care of a specific condition or problem." Medicare stopped recognizing the consult codes in 2010, but the codes didn't disappear from the CPT® book. This chapter will discuss the CPT® definition of consults and how to document and audit them for commercial payers that still recognize consult codes. It will also discuss the correct category of code to report for fee-for-service Medicare patients when a consult is requested.

CPT® added editorial comments to the 2010 edition of the CPT® book, stating that if a transfer of care takes place, the visit should not be billed as a consult. CPT® re-defined a consult, however, as a visit at which the consultant would determine whether to accept the care of the patient for that condition. There are now only two sets of consultation codes: outpatient and office consultations (99241–99245) and inpatient consultations (99251–99255). The 2006 CPT® book deleted confirmatory consultations (99271–99275) and subsequent inpatient consultation visits (99261–99263).

The outpatient/office consult codes (99241–99245) and the inpatient consult codes (99251–99255) can still be used for some commercial insurances and most state Medicaid programs. Medicare HMOs were not required to follow fee-for-service Medicare rules, but most did. This puts the onus on each practice to determine which of its private payers and Medicare Advantage plans still recognize consultations.

Medicare and Consults

What codes will physicians use to bill for services that were consults? For outpatient consults, provided in the office and outpatient department, use new or established patient visit codes: 99241–99245 will be 99201–99215. Review the definition of a new patient from the Centers for Medicare & Medicaid (CMS) manual:

Interpret the phrase "new patient" to mean a patient who has not received any professional services, i.e., E/M service or other face-to-face service (e.g., surgical procedure) from the physician or physician group practice (same physician specialty) within the previous 3 years.

Medicare patients seen in an office or outpatient setting seen at the request of another health care professional for an opinion or advice are reported with office or outpatient codes, new or established patient. Review the rules for new patients and specialty designation in deciding whether to report a new or established patient visit.

Physicians often think that a new problem equals a new patient. This is not true. Whether the patient is seen for a new or existing problem is not a factor in determining if the patient is new. The key driver: If the physician or her same-specialty partner has had a face-to-face professional service with that patient in the past three years. Anywhere. For any reason.

What about consults in the hospital? Admitting physicians must now use modifier AI (capital I, not number 1) on their claim forms to indicate they are the admitting physician when they bill for the admission, 99221–99223. All other physicians who see a patient for the first time in consultation will also bill using the initial hospital care codes (what we call the admission codes 99221–99223). CMS has instructed contractors to pay for multiple initial hospital services for the same patient, even if they are on the same day. For example, a patient may be seen by an internist, a cardiologist and an infectious disease physician on the first day of their hospital stay. For Medicare, all of these physicians would report initial hospital care codes. If the consult service does not meet the requirements for the lowest-level initial hospital service, 99221, (that is, it would have been billed as a 99251 or a 99252), you can bill a Medicare fee-for-service patient for a subsequent hospital visit, even if an initial visit has not been performed. From the *Medicare Claims Processing Manual*, Chapter 12:

Contractors shall not find fault in cases where the medical record appropriately demonstrates that the work and medical necessity requirements are met for reporting a subsequent hospital care code (under the level selected), even though the reported code is for the provider's first E/M service to the inpatient during the hospital stay.

How does a physician bill when she is called to the Emergency Department (ED) to see a fee-for-service Medicare patient who is not admitted? Use the ED codes (99281–99285). Previously, these were billed with outpatient consult codes if the criteria for a consult were met. This means that all physicians of multiple specialties will bill ED codes on the same patient, on the same date of service, perhaps for the same diagnosis.

Consults to observation status fee-for-service Medicare patients should be billed with office and outpatient codes 99201–99215, keeping in mind the definition of a new patient visit. If a patient is in observation status, only the admitting physician uses the observation codes, 99218–99220 or 99234–99236, and these are submitted without a modifier.

Hospitalists also bill the initial hospital services codes for their post-op evaluations for medically necessary, non-surgical management of medical problems. Remember that these services must be medically necessary to manage the patient's medical problems. Post-op services are part of the global surgical package and are part of the single payment paid to the surgeon. The surgeon is responsible for pain management, fluids, nutrition, wound care, and discharge planning.

These codes for fee-for-service Medicare patients do not carry the same requirements as consult codes. These services billed with an office visit code, and Emergency Department code or an initial hospital service code do not require the referring physician NPI number on the claim form. A formal report is not required for Medicare, but CMS notes that the Documentation Guidelines advise physicians who are caring for patients to communicate with one another.

Consults in a nursing facility will be coded with initial nursing facility codes 99304–99306. The admitting physician to a nursing facility will use those codes with an AI modifier. Non-physician practitioners are restricted in their use of these codes.

Consults to Commercial Patients

The medical record of the consulting physician determines whether a service meets the criteria of a consult. The consultation codes require all three of the key components (history, exam and MDM) to meet or exceed the code requirements. CPT notes that the medical record should document the request for the consultation. Consults can be billed using time if the criteria for using time as the determining factor are met. (See the How to Audit Evaluation and Management Services chapter for more on how to use time as the determining factor.)

Outpatient and office consults (99241–99245) do not have new and established patient designations. If the service meets the criteria for a consultation, as defined below, a physician may bill the consultation codes to a patient who is new or established to the practice. Similarly, inpatient consults are for new or established patients. Only one inpatient consultation in the 99251–99255 series may be billed to an individual patient by a physician during the course of a single admission. The patient may have multiple inpatient consults by physicians of different specialties, but each physician may bill only one inpatient consult on that patient during the admission.

In 2006, the AMA deleted two sets of consultation codes from the Evaluation and Management (E/M) series of codes. The confirmatory consults, 99271–99275, were deleted. How should physicians bill for these services now? A patient who presents to the physician office for a second opinion as a *self-referred* patient should be billed using new or established patient visit codes, 99201–99215. A commercially insured patient who is sent to a physician office from another healthcare provider for an opinion (first or second) or evaluation and meets the consult requirements described in this chapter may be billed using the outpatient/office consult codes, 99241–99245.

Subsequent consultation codes, 99261–99263, were also deleted. A consulting physician who provides follow-up inpatient services after an initial inpatient consult should bill subsequent hospital visits, 99231–99233. More than one physician can "round" on a patient in one day, as long as they are of different specialties and the services are medically necessary. Different diagnosis codes help keep these claims from requiring notes before being paid.

What Is a Consult?

A consult is differentiated from a visit by the following factors: The consult is provided by a physician or a non-physician practitioner (NPP) whose opinion or advice is requested from another physician, NPP, or appropriate source. The request and medical necessity for the consult, along with the assessment, are documented in the patient's medical record, and the consultant prepares and sends a written report of the findings to the requesting provider. CPT states that a consult may be requested by another "appropriate source." In reality, the requesting clinician must have a provider number, and that provider number needs to be on the claim form that is submitted for payment.

CPT® added this to its definition of outpatient consults: ". . . for a specific condition or problem or to determine whether to accept responsibility for ongoing management of the patient's entire care or for the care of a specific condition or problem." That gives a physician wide latitude to use the consult codes for visits in order to "determine whether to accept responsibility for ongoing management." Most first-time appointments to a specialty office meet this requirement.

Later in the section, the AMA adds, "Services that constitute a transfer of care (i.e., are provided for the management of the patient's entire care or for the care of a specific condition or problem) are reported with the appropriate new or established. . . ." Some clear examples of this might be:

- A patient is being treated by an oncologist in Florida, and now returns to his first home in Pennsylvania to continue treatment. The oncologist in Florida transfers care of the patient for her treatment to the Pennsylvania physician. An opinion or advice is not being requested.
- A Neurologist sees and diagnoses a patient with multiple sclerosis. The Neurologist does not treat patients with this condition, and refers the patient to another Neurologist at an MS center. The first physician is not requesting an opinion but is transferring care.

Consults still require a request. The request for a consult must be documented in the patient's medical record. The consultant should document this request in the medical record that he prepares. The consultant can receive this request in writing or over the phone. There may be a written order in the medical record when the patient is in the hospital, seen in the ED, or seen in a nursing facility. The request is for an opinion, evaluation, or advice regarding management of a medical problem in order for the service to be a consult. The E/M Documentation Guidelines instruct the requesting physician to document any referrals or consults in the patient's medical record. This supports the level of medical decision making.

The Documentation Guidelines state that referrals or consult requests should be documented in the medical record.

- **DG** *If referrals are made, consultations requested or advice sought, the record should indicate to whom or where the referral or consultation is made or from whom the advice is requested.*

The consultant is required to give an opinion and provide it to the requesting provider. This is a requirement of a consult: **The consultant prepares a report and provides that to the requesting physician.** This can be accomplished in a number of ways:

- The entire report can be in the form of a letter back to the requesting provider.

- A cover letter can be dictated with a copy of the report attached.
- A letter can summarize the findings and recommendations.
- In an Emergency Department or an inpatient or outpatient setting with a shared medical record, the report in the common medical record serves as the report.
- In an office setting in which there is a common medical record, a separate report is prepared and placed in the common medical record. It is advisable that the group has a process by which the report is routed to the requesting physician in some way: via an e-mail notification or by being placed in a separate section of the chart.
- In a shared electronic medical record, the report is sent electronically to the requesting clinician.

The consultant must prepare a report with the results of the evaluation and this must be provided to the requesting provider.

Yes, It's a Consult

Consultants can initiate treatment and order diagnostic tests at the consulting visit, and still bill the patient for a consult. Consults may be billed even when the diagnosis is known by the requesting and consulting physician, prior to the consultation visit. The requesting provider may know the diagnosis but want the expert's opinion to establish an appropriate treatment plan.

Consults can be requested within a group, whether the consultant is the same or a different specialty, *provided* that the service is medically necessary and the service meets the requirements for a consult. Use caution in reporting consultations within a group for the same-specialty physicians. If care is being transferred to a partner, the visit is not a consultation.

Scheduled follow-up services after the initial consult are correctly billed as established patient visits or subsequent hospital visits or subsequent nursing facility visits, depending on the location of the care.

Can a specialist provide and be paid for a second consult on the same patient in the same year? Yes. Remember, these codes are used for new or established patient visits. CPT® does not limit the number of consults a consultant can perform on a single patient in any time period. For example, a Primary Care Physician (PCP) may ask an Orthopedist for an opinion about a patient's chronic and worsening neck pain. The Orthopedist sees the patient, evaluates the problem, and sends a report back to the PCP. No further treatment or follow up is planned by the Orthopedist. Later, the patient returns to the PCP for new onset elbow pain and tenderness. The PCP again sends the patient to the Orthopedist and asks for an opinion. The Orthopedist can bill a consult for this second visit (99241–99245). However, if the patient self-refers back to the Orthopedist for the elbow pain, that visit is correctly billed using established patient visits, 99211–99215.

Some third-party payers will only pay for a single consult to a specific physician on a patient in a year. That is, they would not pay for their subscriber to have a second Orthopedic consultation by the same physician, as described in the preceding paragraph. This is not a CPT® rule, but a payer edit implemented by some third parties.

Here are some statements that meet the requirements for consultations:

"Patient referred by Dr. Wheeler for my evaluation of COPD." Consult performed on an inpatient, with a report in the joint medical record.

"Dear Dr. Primary, thank you for requesting my opinion about Betsy's headaches. I find. . . ." The request is documented, you have rendered an opinion, and the letter serves as a report.

"Dear Dr. Bones, at your request, I have evaluated Ms. Hip's medical condition prior to her surgery. I find her medical problems to be ABC. She is cleared for surgery." The request is documented, you have rendered an opinion, and the letter serves as a report.

"I am seeing this patient at the request of Dr. Ben R. for preoperative medical clearance for osteoarthritis and hypertension. A copy of this report is being returned to Dr. R."

Here are some statements that do *not* meet the requirements for a consult:

"Dear Dr. Primary, thank you for kindly sending me your patient, Betsy, for her headaches." Where is the request for opinion? Can you be sure the PCP has documented it?

"Patient is a 55-year-old male referred to me for treatment of his back pain." This may very well be a consult, but the auditor cannot tell that from this statement. Be clear about whether the patient was sent by another healthcare provider. The report back is not documented.

"Ms. Hip is here prior to her surgery for pre-op clearance." Neither the request nor the returned report is documented. A pre-op may be a consultation, but make sure the auditor can tell that from the documentation. Also, is there medical necessity for the consult?

Only medically necessary services are covered by insurances.

No, It's Not a Consult

If the patient's care is *transferred* to the consultant prior to the first service, the service is *not* a consult. This is new in the CPT® editorial comments in 2010. This situation might occur when a patient is transferred from one hospital to another, and the physician at the second hospital agrees to accept care of the patient prior to the patient's arrival.

Emergency Departments often have a system for referring patients in follow up to primary care doctors or specialists. The ED doctor may provide care on the weekend and ask the patient to call and make an appointment in a physician office the following week, especially for patients who don't have their own doctors. The ED physician is not looking for an opinion from the physician to whom the patient is referred. This encounter would not meet the criteria for a consult.

Patients who self-refer to the practice or who are referred by friends, a nurse in the ED, or relatives, are not considered consults. A patient who moves to the area and establishes care with a new physician is a new patient, not a consult. If there is no order for the consult or no written report, do not bill a consult. Patients who are recalled for annual re-checks are not consults.

I read this in a letter from an Ophthalmologist to a Family Physician. If the FP follows the specialist's advice, the service won't be a consult:

> "Dear Dr. Primary, Ms. Patton had a successful cataract surgery on her left eye on Dec 2, 2005 and is very happy with the result. She wishes to proceed with cataract surgery on her right eye, and this is scheduled for Feb. 2, 2006. I would appreciate a pre-operative evaluation **which may be sent directly to the hospital.**"

If the FP sends the report to the hospital, the visit is not a consult. The report must be sent to the requesting provider, not the hospital or the Ambulatory Surgery Center (ASC).

Pre-Op Evaluations

Consults can be provided for pre-operative clearance for commercial patients. The requirements are the same as for any other consult. Sometimes, the surgeon asks the Primary Care Provider (PCP) to see the patient to provide an opinion about the patient's medical problems prior to surgery. However, be careful about billing and documenting these encounters. If the patient brings a form from a surgery center, this *does not* qualify as a request for opinion from another healthcare provider. These forms rarely provide documentation for an opinion. If the PCP's opinion was requested, make sure that request is documented on the history and physical form, in a letter, or in a report. The PCP should have a request from the surgeon asking for opinion or evaluation. This could be in the form of a request or a copy of the surgeon's note in which the evaluation was ordered.

Also, these pre-op consults must be medically necessary. If the visit is not medically necessary, the physician must inform the patient prior to the delivery of the service that the visit may not be covered by their insurer. The fact that the hospital or ASC mandates a history does not mean that it is medically necessary. Also, some pre-operative E/M services are part of the global payment to the surgeon. Insurers pay for pre-operative evaluation when the patient's condition necessitates this visit. For example, the patient may be elderly, have chronic illnesses, and be on Coumadin. That patient would require medical clearance prior to many surgical procedures.

Whether you are billing a consult or an office visit, be sure to document sufficient history of the present illness. The statement "Patient here for pre-op clearance" does not provide any history of the present illness. Either document the elements of the HPI or the status of the patient's chronic diseases. For example, a physician might document this for an HPI:

> "I am seeing this patient at the request of Dr. Miller for my medical evaluation of the patient prior to her surgery. This patient has had increasing hip pain, loss of mobility, and swelling for the past three years. NSAIDS and PT were unsuccessful in treating the patient's symptoms. Dr. Miller recommended a surgical treatment and the patient agreed. A copy of this evaluation is being sent to Dr. Miller."

Or, an HPI might read:

> "Ms. Jones presents today at the request of Dr. Miller for medical evaluation and clearance prior to her hip surgery. This patient has a history of poorly controlled diabetes, worsening CHF, and a fib. Her medications at present are. . . . The current status of her illnesses . . . A copy of this report, with my recommendations for her medication changes prior to surgery, is being sent to Dr. Miller."

However, even though the consultant documents this request in the HPI, the office should also keep the written request from the requesting provider in the medical record. This could be a form that the requesting provider sends, a letter from the requesting provider, or a copy of the medical note at which the requesting provider recommends for the consult.

Use the diagnosis codes for pre-op clearance as the first diagnosis, the reason for the patient's surgery as the second diagnosis, and the patient's underlying medical problems as the third diagnosis on the claim form. Remember, all services must be medically necessary. The codes for pre-ops are in the V72.81–V72.84 series.

Other Appropriate Source

The AMA has always had a more liberal definition of who can request a consult, describing it as "or other appropriate source." *The CPT® Assistant*, in its July 2002 edition, offers these examples of appropriate sources which, of course, includes physicians: "physician assistants, nurse practitioners, doctor of chiropractic, physical therapist, occupational therapist, speech-language therapist, psychologist, social worker, lawyer or insurance company." However, third-party payers require the NPI number on the claim form. Without that, the claim will not be paid, despite CPT® rules.

Referrals

The CPT® Assistant reminds physicians that the words "referral" and "consultation" are not synonymous. A referral takes place when a patient is sent from Physician A to Physician B (or practitioner) without a request for opinion or evaluation. If there is no request, the service is not a consult, even if Physician B sends a report back to Physician A.

Follow-up Visits to Inpatient Consults

As of January 1, 2006, there were no longer specific codes for follow-up inpatient consultations. If a consultant, subsequent to billing an inpatient consult, provides ongoing care or "follows along" with the requesting physician, bill subsequent hospital visit codes 99231–99233.

Physicians are reluctant to bill for subsequent hospital visits in these situations because they believe that two physicians cannot bill for subsequent hospital visits in the same day. This is only partially true. Two physicians of the same specialty in the same group must bill and be paid as one physician, and so bill one subsequent hospital service in a calendar date. However, physicians from different specialties, providing medically necessary care to the same patient, can both bill and be paid for subsequent hospital visits. If both use the same diagnosis, some contractors may ask for notes, but both medically necessary visits are payable, at least under Medicare's rules. The office may need to appeal an initial denial and send notes from the hospital admission.

Common Misconceptions

Some physicians believe that because they are specialists, all visits are consults. Recently, when auditing some consult visits, I saw a copy of a form that the billing department had sent to a physician. The billing department was questioning whether the service was a consult and asking for the name of the requesting provider. The physician, obviously annoyed at being questioned about his billing, had written in large letters on the form: "I AM THE CONSULTANT!" Unfortunately, the physician was billing consults for follow-up visits he had scheduled with the patient. He may be the consultant, but the visit was not a consultation.

WHY DOES THE OIG CARE?

Now that CMS has eliminated payments for consults, will the Office of Inspector General still care about consults? Probably not. The consult codes have a status indicator of I for Invalid. If you mistakenly submit a claim with consult codes, it will be denied.

Other payers will monitor your use of the consult codes, particularly high-level codes. Commercial payers have compliance departments and will also review records based on an analysis of billing patterns.

RED FLAGS

If you run a report and see no new patient visits—only consults billed to commercial patients—probe some more. Some practices state that they never bill any new patient visits because all patients must be referred into their practice. However, it is the rare practice that allows no patient to self-refer in the course of the year. Or a patient may be referred from the Emergency Department, or from a friend of someone in the practice. These ED referrals do not meet the criteria for a consultation and should be billed as new patient visits.

If you have new providers in your practice, look at a report that shows their use of consult codes. Compare this use with the norms for their specialty and for the established physicians in your office practice. If their use of consult codes varies significantly from long-term providers in the practice, ask why.

Take the time to ask a few providers in your practice to describe the consult rules to you. If you find that they cannot recite them, make auditing consultation services one of your priorities.

Make sure the billing and coding departments have an up-to-date grid that shows which payers still recognize consult codes.

COMPLIANCE SOLUTIONS

New physicians do not always understand the use of consult codes or the billing requirements for a consult. If you have a new physician or NPP in your practice, be sure to educate him on the specific billing requirements for a consultation before you submit claims for these visits.

Meet with new providers and review all of the codes on your encounter form. In a meeting with a new vascular surgeon recently, I asked why he had not billed any codes from the 99241–99245 series. The notes were documented as consults and billed as new patient visits. He showed me the encounter form, on which those codes were labeled as "Outpatient Consults." He said "I can't use those in the office. They're for the outpatient department."

Some specialists bill all of their consults at the same level. I worked with one physician who had received pre-payment requests for notes for five Level 4 outpatient consults, code 99244. The physician's profile got the attention of the contractor because he had billed so many high-level consults. When I asked him what percentage of his consults were billed as Level 4s, he responded "All of them. That's just normal for my specialty." Make sure your providers know what makes a consult, understand the importance of documenting consults properly, and know the basics of the documentation guidelines as they relate to consults. Also, compare the physician profiles, as discussed in the chapter on aberrant billing patterns.

Educating physicians and staff about consults is critical. This is both a revenue and compliance issue for all practices. You do not want to make either of these two mistakes:

1. *Billing services as consults that do not meet the requirements:* This is a huge compliance risk to the provider and the practice. All providers who do consultations need to understand the rules and the documentation requirements.

2. *Never billing a consult, even when one is provided:* Some groups incorrectly stopped billing any consult codes when fee-for-service Medicare stopped recognizing the codes. This costs the practice entitled reimbursement. Think of it as having less money for staff or

benefits. Take the time to learn the rules and feel confident that when you bill for a consult, you have provided and documented that service.

COMPLIANCE PLAN AUDIT SHEET

Auditor Name:	Date of Audit:
Organization Name:	

Consult Audit Sheet **99241–99245 and 99251–99255 Non-Medicare Patients**		
This sheet does not audit for level of service. You can use the entire hospital record, including progress notes and physician orders, as well as the consultation report itself to audit for consults. Letters from other providers can also be used in auditing consult services. ***You must answer YES to questions 1–4.***		
Answer yes or no to the following questions by checking the appropriate box/circle:		
1. Is there documentation in the requesting or consulting provider's medical record asking for a consult?	☐ Yes	◯ No
2. Is the reason for the consult documented?	☐ Yes	◯ No
3. Was a report generated?	☐ Yes	◯ No
4. Is there evidence that a copy of the report or a letter with the physician opinion was sent to the requesting provider?	☐ Yes	◯ No
You must answer NO to questions 5–8 to bill for a consultation for all payers.		
5. Was the patient self-referred?	☐ Yes	◯ No
6. Was the patient's care transferred to you prior to you seeing the patient?	☐ Yes	◯ No
7. Was the patient's visit to your office part of regularly scheduled follow up to your office?	☐ Yes	◯ No
8. Was the service performed as part of a standing order in the medical record?	☐ Yes	◯ No

CHAPTER 6

Critical Care Services

Critical care services are defined as care of critically ill or injured patients who require constant physician attention. In these patients, there is a high probability of sudden, clinically significant, or life-threatening deterioration, which requires the highest level of physician preparedness to intervene urgently. To bill for critical care time, the physician must be in the same location as the patient and immediately available to provide patient care. The physician may bill only for providing critical care services to a single patient during any one-time period. As with all services, critical care must be medically necessary and reasonable. Although critical care is often provided on an emergency basis, this is not a requirement for critical care.

Here are some characteristics of critical care services:

- Often involve single or multiple vital system failure or trauma.
- May require extensive interpretation of multiple databases and advanced technology.
- Requires highly complex medical decision making.
- The physician is providing critical care interventions.
- Usually but not always performed in a critical care area.

Not only must the patient's condition be critical, the physician must also be providing treatment. If the patient is dying, but intervention is stopped, it is no longer critical care by the CPT® definition.

Here is how the Centers for Medicare & Medicaid Services (CMS) *Internet-Only Manual* defines a critically ill patient and critical care:

> *Critical care is defined as the direct delivery by a physician(s) of medical care for a critically ill or critically injured patient. A critical illness or injury acutely impairs one or more vital organ systems such that there is a high probability of imminent or life-threatening deterioration in the patient's condition.*
>
> *Critical care involves high complexity decision making to assess, manipulate, and support vital system functions(s) to treat single or multiple vital organ system failure and/or to prevent further life-threatening deterioration of the patient's condition.*

Examples of vital organ system failure include, but are not limited to: central nervous system failure, circulatory failure, shock, renal, hepatic, metabolic, and/or respiratory failure. Although critical care typically requires interpretation of multiple physiologic parameters and/or application of advanced technology(s), critical care may be provided in life-threatening situations when these elements are not present.

Providing medical care to a critically ill, injured, or post-operative patient qualifies as a critical care service only if both the illness or injury and the treatment being provided meet the above requirements.

When billing critical care services, count the time spent performing these services:
- Working on the patient's case at the bedside or on the floor.
- Devoting complete attention to the patient.
- Discussing the case with other specialists while on the critical care unit and immediately available to the patient.
- Discussing the case with the patient's family while on the unit and immediately available to the patient, *if* the patient is unable to make his own decisions at that time *and* the discussion is necessary to obtain relevant clinical history or to discuss treatment decisions.
- Reviewing data while on the unit and immediately available to the patient.
- Obtaining necessary clinical historical data from patient's family if the patient is unable to provide the history.
- Performing procedures bundled into critical care.
- Conducting clinical recordkeeping and writing orders.
- Discussing the case with medical and nursing staff.

Do not include time spent in these activities in critical care time:
- Discussing the case or giving verbal orders via the phone while off the unit.
- Reviewing the literature.
- Providing E/M services to any other patient.
- Explaining the patient's condition to the family. Both CPT® and CMS specifically note that updating the patient's family may not be included in critical care time.
- Performing procedures that are not bundled into critical care services.
- If billing for a non-bundled procedure, do not count that the time spent in performing the procedure in your critical care time.

The *Internet-Only Manual* emphasizes the importance of documenting the physician's time and availability to care for the patient as a condition for billing for critical care services:

> *The duration of critical care time to be reported is the time the physician spent working on the critical care patient's case, whether that time was spent at the immediate bedside or elsewhere on the floor, but immediately available to the patient.*

Location

Critical care typically is provided in the critical care unit but may be provided elsewhere. The patient's condition and the services provided define critical care, not the location of the service. Sometimes, patients are admitted to a telemetry unit because no other bed is available. In those cases, it would be inappropriate to bill critical care based solely on the patient's location. Also, patients admitted to a critical care unit solely for nursing observation or because hospital policy requires it for administration of certain drugs should not be billed as critical care.

When the patient is well enough to be transferred from the critical care unit, it usually indicates that the patient is no longer critically ill. The note might read, "Patient can be transferred to the floor this morning." Bill for a subsequent hospital visit at whatever level is required, performed, and documented.

Billing Requirements

The time spent providing critical care services must be recorded in the hospital medical record. Time spent over the course of a 24-hour period can be added together. The time does not need to be continuous. Here are some other rules:

- Regarding Emergency Department (ED) visits and critical care, a single physician cannot bill for critical care services and an ED visit on the same day for the same patient. An ED visit and critical care are never payable on the same day. If the patient is critical in the ED, bill only the critical care codes.
- If you see a patient in the morning and provide a subsequent hospital visit and the patient becomes critically ill later in the day, you can bill for the critical care service later in the day. Attach a 25 modifier on the subsequent hospital visit and send the notes with the claim.

- You may also bill for a subsequent hospital visit performed later in the day, after a critical care service, if the patient is no longer critical. Again, attach a 25 modifier to the subsequent hospital visit, document the critical care time, and submit the notes with the claim.
- Be prepared to send the critical care notes with all claims. Make sure that time, medical necessity, and the treatment provided are documented in all encounters. The note must be legible.
- If the critical care services total fewer than 30 minutes, bill an E/M service. This would typically be a subsequent hospital visit.
- Remember, you cannot provide services to any other patient while billing for critical care time. If the physician is called away to care for another patient, do not count that time toward the critical care time. Critical care requires a physician's *full* attention.
- Time does not need to be continuous. Add together all of the time on each calendar date.
- Do not bill 99292 alone for any day; it is an add-on code and must be billed after 99291 is billed.
- Only one physician may bill for any one time period. It is common for one physician to see a patient early in the day and provide critical care services and a partner of the same specialty in the same group may see the patient in the evening. In order for the second physician to report the add on code 99292, the first physician must have met the full 74 minute time threshold for the initial critical care.

Procedures Performed While Providing Critical Care Services

Certain procedures are bundled into critical care and may not be billed separately. When the physician is providing the following bundled services, the time performing them may be included in the time counted as critical care, according to both CMS and CPT®:

The following services when performed on the day a physician bills for critical care are included in the critical care service and should not be reported separately:

- *The interpretation of cardiac output measurements (CPT® 93561, 93562);*
- *Chest x-rays, professional component (CPT® 71010, 71015, 71020);*
- *Blood gases, and information data stored in computers (e.g., ECGs, blood pressures, hematologic data-CPT® 99090);*

- *Gastric intubation (CPT® 43752, 43753);*
- *Pulse oximetry (CPT® 94760, 94761, 94762);*
- *Temporary transcutaneous pacing (CPT® 92953);*
- *Ventilator management (CPT® 94002–94004, 94660, 94662); and*
- *Vascular access procedures (CPT® 36000, 36410, 36415, 36591, 36600).*

Any other procedures may be billed separately. However, the time spent performing separately billed, unbundled procedures may *not* be counted in the critical care time.

Multiple Physicians Providing Critical Care on a Single Day

Physicians from different specialties may provide medically necessary critical care services on the same day, but not for the same time period. Only one physician "shall bill for critical care services during any one single period of time." CMS clarified this policy in Transmittal 1548 released Jan. 9, 2008. Typically, when physicians of different specialties are seeing the same critically ill patient, they are addressing different problems and will use different diagnosis codes.

Physicians from the same practice, of the same specialty, should bill for critical care services "as if they were one physician." This may happen when one physician leaves work for the day and another comes in to care for the patient. Within a group, physicians of the same specialty should bill 99291 only once in a day. Subsequent time by that physician or the covering physician should be billed with 99292.

The CMS manual addresses services by more than one physician of the same specialty and group:

*The initial critical care time, billed as CPT® code 99291, must be met by a **single** physician **or qualified NPP**. This may be performed in a single period of time or be cumulative **by the same physician** on the same calendar date. A history or physical exam performed by one group partner for another group partner in order for the second group partner to make a medical decision would not represent critical care services.*

After the initial 74 minutes have been met, however: *The service [99292] may represent aggregate time met by a single physician **or physicians** in the same group practice with the same medical specialty in order to meet the duration of minutes required for CPT® code 99292. The aggregated critical care visits must be medically necessary and each aggregated visit must meet the definition of critical care in order to combine the times.*

When multiple physicians are caring for a critically ill patient, each must be managing one or more illnesses or injuries. If an Intensivist is managing the patient's illness, it may not be medically necessary for a hospitalist to attend to the patient on the same day.

Billing Within a Group

Third-party payers and Medicare use specialty designation as an edit when paying claims. Each physician should be enrolled with her correct specialty.

Medicare instructs carriers to pay physicians within the same group of a single specialty as if the services were provided by a single physician. Physicians of different specialties within the same group can bill and be paid without regard to being part of a single group. Physicians from the same group but different specialties bill for critical care services, with both using the initial critical care code, 99291, to indicate 30–74 minutes of critical care services. For example, if an Intensivist and a Cardiologist both see a patient in the critical care unit and provide medically necessary services on the same day, both can bill and be paid. Each physician should bill for the critical care services provided. Be sure that the physicians are enrolled in the Medicare program under the correct specialty. Their documentation must reflect both the time spent on services and the medical necessity for both visits.

Two physicians of the same specialty and same group would bill for the services as if one physician had provided the service. If a physician sees a critically ill patient for a total time of 105 minutes, he would bill 99291–1 unit, and 99292–1 unit. If Physician A sees the patient for 74 minutes and Physician B, a partner of the same specialty and *same* group, sees the patient in the same day for 31 minutes, they submit the claim the same way: 99291–1 unit and 99292–1 unit. Remember that the first physician must fully meet the time requirement for 99291 before additional critical care may be billed by a partner. The CMS reference for this is above, in the section on billing for multiple physicians providing care in the same day.

Physicians from the same group but different specialties each bill for their critical care services using the initial critical care code, 99291, to indicate 30–74 minutes of critical care services.

Non-Physician Practitioners

Non-physician practitioners (NPPs) may provide and bill for critical care, but critical care may not be billed as a shared service. The critical care reported may not be a combination of physician and NPP time. Care provided by the physician or the NPP in a group are both payable, but not on the same day. The group essentially needs to choose to bill either the physician time or the NPP time for a given date of service. In most groups, it would be the physician time. The group may not add together the time of the NPP and the physician and report that.

The CMS manual states that shared services (services provided jointly by a physician and an NPP) may not be applied to critical care billing. Here is the citation:

> *A split/shared E/M service performed by a physician and a qualified NPP of the same group practice (or employed by the same employer) cannot be reported as a critical care service. Critical care services are reflective of the care and management of a critically ill or critically injured patient by an individual physician or qualified non-physician practitioner for the specified reportable period of time.*

> *Unlike other E/M services where a split/shared service is allowed the critical care service reported shall reflect the evaluation, treatment and management of a patient by an individual physician or qualified non-physician practitioner and shall not be representative of a combined service between a physician and a qualified NPP.*

> *When CPT® code time requirements for both 99291 and 99292 and critical care criteria are met for a medically necessary visit by a qualified NPP the service shall be billed using the appropriate individual NPI number. Medically necessary visit(s) that do not meet these requirements shall be reported as subsequent hospital care services.*

Teaching Physician Rules

Report only the time spent by the attending or teaching physician for critical care services. Residents' and interns' time may not be added to the attending physician's time. The resident's note may be used to support the nature of the patient's illness and the intensive nature of the interventions provided. However, the teaching physician must personally be present for all of the time reported on the claim form. The teaching physician must document substantive information about the patient's condition, that she participated in the patient's care, and the time that she personally spent in critical care treatment. Then, she may tie her notes to the resident's note.

Family Meetings

CPT® and CMS rules related to family meetings for critically ill patients are the same. Time spent with the family may not be counted for updating the family on the patient's condition. Family meetings may only be counted in two cases: 1) when the patient is unable to participate in giving a history and/or making decisions about his care and 2) when the discussion is necessary for deciding on treatment. The physician should document that the patient is unable to participate in providing the history or making decisions, the necessity for the discussion, and the treatment decisions that were needed. A summary of this should be included in the medical record.

Post-Op Critical Care

Medicare instructs carriers to pay for post-op critical care *only* when the care is unrelated to the surgical service. If the patient's condition is a result of the surgery, Medicare will *not* pay for critical care services. If the patient's condition is unrelated, e.g., a patient becomes critically ill from heart failure after a hip replacement, that service is payable. Surgeons treating a trauma patient may sometimes bill for critical care in the post op period. For example, the surgeon operates on the spleen, but also is treating a cranial crush injury.

Critical Care and a Procedure on the Same Day

A physician may be asked to perform a procedure on the same day that she provides critical care service. For example, the physician may introduce a tunneled catheter on the same day as she provides critical care. This procedure is not bundled into 99291/99292, so the physician may bill for it separately. (Be sure that the time spent in performing the procedure is not included in the critical care time.) This procedure has a 10-day global period. When billing it, attach a 25 modifier on the critical care service. Use the diagnosis for the catheter placement that best represents the reason for the catheter placement (need for high-risk medications, malnutrition, etc.) and use a different diagnosis code for the critical care, such as respiratory failure or kidney failure. Although a different diagnosis is not needed on the day of the procedure, because you are using the 25 modifier, it will be needed for subsequent critical care days to be paid. The catheter insertion has a 10-day global period, so subsequent critical care days need to be billed with a 24 modifier to indicate that the E/M service is not related to the procedure and needs a diagnosis code to justify the service. Of course, if the procedure is the only service performed, do not bill critical care or an E/M.

Critical Care and Another E/M Service on the Same Day

Critical care may be provided on the same day as a distinct and separate E/M service if the two services represent two distinct episodes of care. If the patient is critically ill from the start of the episode of care, bill only for critical care. For example, a patient presents to the hospital and is admitted with fever, shortness of breath, and abnormal white count. The patient is sick but not critical, and is admitted to a medical floor. Three hours later, the patient becomes hypoxic and goes into septic shock. The physician would bill for both services: the initial hospital service with 25 modifier, and critical care. Two separate notes would support that the services were distinct. However, if the physician arrived in the Emergency Department and found the patient in critical condition, report only the critical care codes, even though the documentation is a dictated history and physical.

Examples of Documenting Time in Critical Care

CPT® requires that total time spent in critical care services is documented in the medical record. CMS also requires total time, not start and stop time, but states that for each date and entry, time should be documented. If a physician sees the patient multiple times in a day, instead of documenting the time at the last visit, document time each time an entry is made into the medical record, and add together the time in the calendar date.

> "Critical care time—50 minutes."
> "Critical care time spent at this visit—1 hour, 20 minutes."
> "I spent 1 hour of critical care time. Time spent doing procedures not included in this time."
> "Time spent doing procedures—30 minutes. Time spent in critical care—45 minutes."

Many physicians want us to assume their total critical care time based on the running time entries they make as they document the day's activities. However, there is no way of knowing from that running log if the physician spent time off the unit or providing care to other patients. The only way to bill critical care is to document, using one of the above examples, the total time spent on the calendar date. Avoid abbreviating time, such as "cc 45'."

RED FLAGS

Here are some of the red flags that could set off warning bells for your carrier about critical care billing:

- Critical care billed for an excessive number of consecutive days. Bill a single patient only for consecutive days of critical care if the patient remains in critical condition and you are providing treatment. These situations will often trigger a request for notes. When the patient is stable, do not bill critical care, even if the patient is still in the unit. The last day the patient is in intensive care before being transferred to a medical floor, the patient is often not critically ill.

- Multiple dates of service in which an E/M service was billed along with critical care. There are a few instances in which you can bill an E/M service and critical care for the same patient on the same day. One is if the patient is not critical in the morning and a subsequent visit is made, and the patient becomes critically ill later in the day. If your billing pattern shows this combination often, inquire. Do your physicians understand the rules for billing both situations?

- Billing for critical care and a discharge visit on the same day. If the patient is well enough to go home, bill only the discharge visit. If the patient dies or is transferred to another facility and the requirements for critical care are met, bill only the critical care.

- Diagnosis codes that do not indicate how sick the patient is. The diagnosis codes on the insurance form should reflect the severity of the patient's illness or disease. If they don't, question if the diagnosis code is wrong or if the service provided would have been more appropriately billed with non-critical care codes.

- Excessive total amount of critical care time. Are you billing for an unrealistic or unusual amount of time given the number of hours in a day or number of hours the physician was at the hospital? If your ICU shift is 8 hours long, it is unlikely that you would have spent the entire 8 hours doing critical care. Some of the activities of the day would probably be for services not included in critical care time.

- A patient who requires many hours of critical care in a day.

Take the time to look at your critical care billing in the above areas.

COMPLIANCE SOLUTIONS

When I audit records for hospital services, the error rate is always significantly higher than for office visit services. And when I audit critical care services, the error rate is higher than for other hospital services. There are three problems that I routinely find:

- The patient's condition does not seem to be critical;
- The patient's condition is critical, but treatment is stopped except for comfort measures; and
- Time is not documented.

If your practice provides and bills for critical care services, include this area in your audit this year. The good news is this: physicians are remarkably consistent in their documentation and billing habits and practices. You only need to look at two or three critical care notes per physician. The audit is not difficult. If you need to, take a clinician with you for an afternoon of auditing in the Health Information Department, to help with the decision about whether the patient's condition is critical. Then, look for time. If time is not documented in the medical record on the day that you bill 99291, you cannot bill for critical care.

If you find that time is not documented, immediately, re-educate your physicians. If you have collected government funds to which you were not entitled, these must be returned.

COMPLIANCE PLAN AUDIT SHEET

Auditor Name:	Date of Audit:
Organization Name:	

Critical Care Services
To perform this audit you will need: • Medical record for each critical care service • Copy of the CMS-1500 form, if submitted, or billing codes selected by the provider Select 10 services for each provider for whom codes 99291–99292 were billed.

Answer yes or no to the following questions by checking the appropriate box/circle:

Is total time spent documented in the medical note?	☐ Yes	○ No
Is the patient's condition critical?	☐ Yes	○ No
Were intervention and treatment of an intensive nature documented?	☐ Yes	○ No
If 99292 (an add-on code) is billed, is 99291 billed the same day as well?	☐ Yes	○ No
Is 99291 billed only once each day for all physicians in the same group, same specialty?	☐ Yes	○ No
If a procedure was performed that is separately billable, can you tell if the times was subtracted from the critical care?	☐ Yes	○ No

You must answer yes to these questions to bill for critical care.

CHAPTER 7

Billing for 99211

The lowest-level established patient office visit has been called "the most abused code in the CPT® book." It seems astonishing that a low-level code, commonly referred to as a nurse visit, could be considered in this way, but astonishing only until you consider two things:

- The high volume of 99211 visits billed to Medicare and other third-party payers in the course of a year; and
- The propensity of medical practices to add 99211 when billing for another service by nursing staff.

If you listen to advice from so-called experts, you'll hear that you should "always" bill 99211 in certain situations or "never" bill it in those very same situations. It's no wonder that physicians and their staffs are confused.

The national, non-facility payment for 99211 in the first three months of 2015 is $20.02. To look up national and local payment amounts on CMS's website, go to https://www.cms.gov/apps/physician-fee-schedule/search/search-criteria.aspx

99211 Defined

99211 is the lowest-level, established patient visit code. The CPT® book defines it as:

> *Office or other outpatient visit for the evaluation and management of an established patient that may not require the presence of a physician. Usually, the presenting problem(s) are minimal. Typically, 5 minutes are spent performing or supervising these services.*

This describes a face-to-face service (not a phone call) with the physician, non-physician practitioner (NPP), or, more typically, a member of the physician's staff with an established patient. The definition notes that the patient's presenting problem is usually minimal. As you read the definition, however, you notice something is missing from the descriptions for the other E/M codes: the level of history, exam, and medical decision making that is required to document a 99211. This lack of specific definition is one of the problems with deciding when you can and cannot bill the code. It is clear from the definition that the visit does not require a physician or NPP to see the patient in order to bill for the service.

Bill a 99211 only when there is no other CPT® code that more accurately describes that day's services, such as a venipuncture or injection. Do not bill 99211 in lieu of billing another service. Do not automatically bill 99211 with another service such as an allergy shot administration.

Nurse visits provided to Medicare patients are always incident to services. Be sure to review the chapter in this book on incident to services if you are providing nurse visits to Medicare patients.

Medical Necessity

The first requirement for all services is medical necessity. Neither Medicare nor any third party will pay for a service unless the patient's condition requires the service. Specifically, office policy does not constitute medical necessity. Some practices say, "It's our policy that all patients who receive an allergy injection also have a nurse visit to evaluate the patient." This policy does not constitute medical necessity or accurate coding.

Some patients receiving allergy injections may require a nurse visit at the time of the procedure, based on their complaints at the time of the visit. But for many patients, the administration of the allergen is the only medically necessary service. And remember, the payment for the administration of the allergy is your payment. This includes assessing the patient prior to giving the injection and after.

The CPT® Assistant specifically stated in April 2005 that it was not correct coding to bill for a nurse visit when the purpose of the visit is vaccine administration only. Some patients get behind on their scheduled immunizations and come in for immunizations only. Report only the vaccine administration code and the vaccine, if purchased by the practice. Do not report 99211 in addition. The CPT® Assistant noted that the payment for the administration includes administrative staff services such as preparing the chart and clinical staff services including taking routine vital signs, obtaining a vaccine history, presenting the vaccine permission form, preparing and administering the vaccine, and observing for any reaction.

Separate from Other Services

Billing a 99211 when you provide any other service requires that the service provided is separate from other services provided that day. For example, if you have a patient who comes to the office for a venipuncture or a flu shot, it's incorrect to bill the patient for a nurse visit. Some practices say, "My nurse always evaluates the patient when we a) take their blood, b) give them an allergy shot, or c) or give a flu shot. Remember that the documentation for the 99211 must reflect both the medical necessity for the visit and the distinct, separate service that was provided.

Some contractors give specific examples of when not to bill 99211. For instance, a patient comes in for a lab service. The blood is drawn. The nurse calls the patient later in the day with the results and instructs the patient to adjust his medication. Bill only for the lab service, not for a 99211. No face-to-face service occurred to perform the evaluation and management component of the service, and you may not use 99211 to bill for telephone calls.

Coumadin Clinics

Many practices have developed Coumadin clinics and bill an E/M service for managing patients on Coumadin. You must establish medical necessity first to bill these services. Although physicians tell us that the literature supports the assertion that closer management leads to better outcomes, the contractors have not always agreed that this translates into paying for all patients to attend Coumadin clinics.

It is never a Medicare billable service if the E/M component takes place over the phone. An example of this is if the patient has his blood drawn early in the day and a staff member calls the patient later to report the results and adjust the patient's dosage.

The service is payable if the nurse, with the lab results available, has a face-to-face service with the patient, takes a brief history, discusses the results and dosage with the physician who is in the office at the time, and adjusts the patient's medicines. Under Medicare, this encounter would be billed incident to the physician. Keep in mind that the contractor must consider each of these services to be medically necessary. Some groups bill a nurse visit if the patient's treatment changes, because that shows medical necessity. If the patient's dosage remains the same, they do not bill a nurse visit.

99211 and Injections

The *Internet-Only Manual* tells practices that they may not use 99211 to report a service that is more accurately described as an injection. Also, injections are not payable on the same day as a nurse visit. From the CMS manual:

> *For services furnished on or after January 1, 2004, do not allow payment for CPT® code 99211, with or without modifier 25, if it is billed with a nonchemotherapy drug infusion code or a chemotherapy administration code. Apply this policy to code 99211 when it is billed with a diagnostic or therapeutic injection code on or after January 1, 2005.*

Simply, if a Medicare patient comes into the office solely for the purpose of receiving an injection, do not bill a 99211 instead of the injection.

99211 as an Incident to Service

For Medicare patients, 99211 performed by a staff member is an incident to service. A nurse, medical assistant, or other employee of the physician must make sure the service meets the incident to requirements to bill—and they would be limited to billing only 99211. In summary, these requirements are:

- Patient is an established patient.
- The problem is an established problem for which the physician has initiated treatment.
- The treatment is an integral part of the patient's service.
- The physician remains involved in the patient's care.
- The physician (or another supervising physician) is in the office, immediately available to the nurse and patient. Report the service under the provider number of the physician who is in the office, supervising.
- The employee providing the service is an employee, contracted staff member, or leased staff member of the physician or the group that employs the physician. The employee's expense must be an expense to the physician practice.

A Quick Recap

To bill 99211:

- It must be a medically necessary service;
- It must not be in lieu of billing another, more accurately described service;
- The patient must be an established patient;
- There must be a face-to-face service;

- The date of service and legible identity of the provider is documented; and
- For Medicare, the service must meet incident to rules.

Do not bill 99211:
- If all you did was provide an injection or drew blood;
- For renewing a prescription;
- For making phone calls;
- For services performed solely as part of an office policy; or
- If all of the documentation for the service is on a flow sheet for another service.

Clinical Examples

The most common example of a 99211, nurse visit, is for a patient who requires a periodic blood pressure check. A patient with hypertension, high cholesterol, and diabetes presents at the office for regular follow up. The patient brings his home blood pressure readings in for review. These show the patient's blood pressure to be in poor control. On exam, the patient's blood pressure is noted to be 150/90.

The physician adjusts the patient's medications and asks the patient to return to the office once each week for the next five weeks for a blood pressure check, and to return to see the physician in six weeks. The physician documents the plan in the chart and asks the patient to make the follow-up appointments. In each of the next five weeks, the patient returns to the office, the nurse takes the patient's blood pressure, takes a brief history, documents the presence or absence of any side effects, and notes the medication dosage in the chart. If the patient's blood pressure is not good, the nurse may consult the physician and note the new orders/advice from the physician in the plan.

The above service meets the 99211 criteria because:
- It was a medically necessary service.
- It meets all of the criteria for an incident to service. (The incident to rule is a Medicare rule, not a commercial rule.)
- The service was provided face to face.
- No other CPT® code more accurately describes the service performed.
- The physician was in the office when the service was provided.
- The employee who provided the service is an expense to the practice.

Documentation

What documentation is required by the nursing staff member? The extent of the note will depend on the severity of the presenting problem and status of the patient. However, keep in mind that the typical presenting problem for a 99211 is minimal, so the documentation need not be extensive. The nurse should document:

- Date of service;
- The reason for the visit;
- Any side effects of treatment or illness;
- Relevant physical findings, such as BP;
- Plan; and
- Name of person providing the service.

It looks like a lot of bullet points, but here's how it translates into a short note:

DOS: The patient is here today for a BP check. BP was high at last MD visit. No problems with medicines. No dizziness or other problems at home. BP today is 138/76. Looks well. Discussed with MD. No change in meds. Return in 1 week for another check. Signed.

WHY DOES THE OIG CARE?

In a word, the Office of Inspector General (OIG) cares because of *volume*. The huge volume of services Medicare pays means that even with a relatively low level of payment, it represents a lot of healthcare dollars. The national, non-facility rate for 99211 is less than $20.

Doctors have seen this code as an opportunity to increase their revenues without spending their own time. The practice can bill for staff time. Since physician time is the most valued and limited resource in the practice, the ability to bill for staff time can significantly enhance revenue.

If you do a search in any major search engine on billing for 99211, you'll find conflicting advice, sometimes within the same article. Some consultants or physicians advocate billing 99211 with every allergy injection, for example. Others caution against doing so. This confusion about whether or not to bill a 99211 with a specific service and how to document the service when provided, makes billing the code fertile ground for the OIG.

RED FLAGS

Certain billing patterns will raise the concerns of contractors. Review your billing patterns and office policies and be on the lookout for:

- A pattern of billing 99211 with another code, such as venipuncture, flu shot, allergy injection.
- An office policy that mandates billing a nurse visit with another type of service.
- Billing 99211 and a J code together. This is a sign that you were billing 99211 in place of the injection code.
- Higher frequency of nurse visits billed to Medicare than typical for your specialty.
- Documentation for the service is entirely noted on a flow sheet for another service.

COMPLIANCE SOLUTIONS

Remember, if your self-audit reveals significant errors, consult your attorney. You are required to return to Medicare any monies paid to you that you are not entitled to receive.

Review your office policies. If you have a policy in place that states that you "always" bill a 99211 with another service, revise the policy with these rules in mind. Pay special attention to the issue of medical necessity. Services must be medically necessary to that particular patient on that specific date of service.

Instruct your nurses to document their nurse visits using the model described on the previous pages. Documentation on a flow sheet alone may not be sufficient in all cases and is less likely to show medical necessity. Be sure the code you use for services, such as injections, venipuncture, etc., is the accurate code for the service and that you are not billing a 99211 in place of another service.

If your E/M coding profile shows a higher frequency of 99211s than is usual for your specialty, be sure to look carefully at your billing practices and documentation. A coding profile that varies from the CMS expected can trigger audit requests, although such a pattern may be completely justified by your care and documentation.

COMPLIANCE PLAN AUDIT SHEET

Auditor Name:	Date of Audit:
Organization Name:	

Billing for 99211		
For **Medicare patients**, you must also answer all the incident to questions to bill this service. There are two issues to consider: Is the service medically necessary and is that medical necessity adequately documented?		
Do you "always" bill a 99211 with another service, without answering the question of medical necessity? Use caution if this is your policy.		
*You must answer **YES** to the next three of questions to bill this code:*		
Answer yes or no to the following questions by checking the appropriate box/circle:		
Is there a note in the progress note section of the chart? (Do not count notes on flow sheets.)	☐ Yes	◯ No
Was the service being billed a face-to-face service?	☐ Yes	◯ No
Can you determine a reason for the visit, and does it seem medically necessary?	☐ Yes	◯ No

Use **caution** if these statements are true:
"We always bill a nurse visit with an allergy injection/venipuncture/B-12 shot because our nurse always does an independent assessment."
"It's our policy to bill a nurse visit whenever the nurse pulls the chart and sees the patient."

CHAPTER 8

Incident to Billing and Shared Visits

What are incident to services and how are they paid? The incident to provision is a Medicare billing rule dating to the early days of the program in the 1960s. The rule allows the physician practice to bill for services provided by a staff member or a non-physician practitioner under the national provider identifier (NPI) of the physician It also allows a practice to report services provided by a staff member under the provider number of a non-physician practitioner.

Incident to billing means billing for a service provided by someone who is not the physician *as if* the physician had performed the service. That is, the claim is submitted to Medicare with the physician's provider name and number and with no indication to the carrier that the service was provided by anyone else. Medicare pays the claim at 100% of the physician fee schedule.

Incident to billing is a Medicare billing rule. Commercial payers set their own rules about billing for NPPs and staff members in the physician office. This chapter will discuss the rules for incident to billing and for shared visits, both Medicare rules.

Here's how the *Medicare Carriers Manual* describes this type of billing:

> *Incident to a physician's professional services means that the services or supplies are furnished as an integral, although incidental, part of the physician's personal professional services in the course of diagnosis or treatment of an injury or illness.*

Incident to services, then, are part of a physician-initiated treatment plan provided by a member of the physician's staff. The services are billed under the physician's name and provider number, as if the physician provided the services. Incident to billing is allowed in the physician office. A practice may not bill incident to services in a facility, such as an outpatient department, inpatient department, or in a nursing home.

There are two common situations in which incident to services are billed. One is a nurse visit or service in which a nurse or medical assistant is the only staff member who sees the patient that day. These visits may only be billed at the 99211 level. The second common situation is when an NPP sees the patient as part of the physician's plan of care. These NPP visits in the office, when they meet incident to requirements, may be billed as if the physician performed the service, allowing the practice to collect at 100% of the physician fee schedule amount. If the NPP bills the service under his or her own provider number, the practice collects 85% of the physician fee schedule amount.

After an absence from the Work Plan since 2004, incident to billing reappears in 2007 and again in 2012. In August 2009, the Office of Inspector General (OIG) released a report called "Prevalence and Qualifications of Non-physicians Who Performed Medicare Physician Services." The shocking results will be described later in this chapter.

Incident to services were back on the OIG Work Plan in 2012. Whether these services are on or off the Work Plan in the current year, practices should pay attention to these rules.

Physicians: Incident-To Services (New)

We will review physician billing for "incident-to" services to determine whether payment for such services had a higher error rate than that for non-incident-to services. We will also assess CMS's ability to monitor services billed as "incident-to." Medicare Part B pays for certain services billed by physicians that are performed by nonphysicians incident to a physician office visit. A 2009 OIG review found that when Medicare allowed physicians' billings for more than 24 hours of services in a day, half of the services were not performed by a physician. We also found that unqualified nonphysicians performed 21 percent of the services that physicians did not perform personally. Incident-to services represent a program vulnerability in that they do not appear in claims data and can be identified only by reviewing the medical record. They may also be vulnerable to overutilization and expose Medicare beneficiaries to care that does not meet professional standards of quality. Medicare's Part B coverage of services and supplies that are performed incident to the professional services of a physician is in the Social Security Act, § 1861(s) (2)(A). Medicare requires providers to furnish such information as may be necessary to determine the amounts due to receive payment. (Social Security Act, § 1833(e).) (OEI; 00–00–00000; expected issue date: FY 2013; new start)

A quick style note: The OIG uses incident-to with a hyphen, and the Centers for Medicare & Medicaid Services (CMS) omits the hyphen for incident to services. I have elected to follow CMS's style and omit the hyphen.

Key Medicare Incident to Billing Requirements

To bill incident to, the following requirements must be met:

1. The service must be an "integral, although incidental, part of the physician's professional services."
2. The physician must be directly supervising the service. That is, the physician must be in the suite of offices at the time the service is performed, immediately available to provide assistance if needed. This provision is strictly enforced. If the physician is in the car between the hospital and the office, on vacation, or anywhere but in the office, you may not bill the service as incident to. If the treating physician in a group practice is out of the office, but a partner is available, bill the service under the billing number of the supervising physician who is in the office at the time the service was performed. "In the suite of offices" is commonly interpreted as offices that are not separated by a stairwell or elevator.
3. The physician must perform "an initial service and subsequent services of a frequency which reflect his/her active participation in and management of the course of treatment." Stated another way, the physician must see the patient first—at a previous visit—and establish the treatment plan. It is this provision that many interpret to mean the physician must see the patient for any new problems. Because the service must be part of the physician's plan of care, new problems can never be billed incident to, billed under the physician's NPI. The NPP can see the patient for a new problem but must bill the service under her own provider number.

   How does a practice show that the physician has stayed involved with the plan of care? Some practices have a policy that the physician and NPP alternate visits. Some NPPs document the visit in their notes and that the treatment plan was discussed with the physician. The physician can review the documentation and add any comments to the note. The chart should show evidence that the physician has stayed involved in the plan of care.
4. The service being provided must be an expense to the physician or the physician practice. The NPP or staff member providing the care must be an employee of the physician, an employee of the group that employs the physician, or a leased or contracted employee of the physician practice.

5. Incident to services may only be performed in the physician office or patient's home. They are usually performed in the physician office. In the rare circumstance when both the physician and practice-employed nurse are visiting the patient in his own home, you can bill for services the nurse performs, such as an injection. You may not bill if the nurse visits the patient without the presence of the physician. You may not perform incident to services in the hospital or nursing home.

New patients can never be billed as incident to. The very nature of incident to services is that the service is part of the physician's plan of care. It would be impossible for a non-physician practitioner to bill a new patient as part of the physician's plan of care; the physician must see the patient at a *prior* visit to establish the plan, not during the initial visit.

Who Can Bill Their Services Incident to?

Employees, leased employees, and independent contractors of the physician or group that employs the physician can bill their services incident to the physician services and use the physician's name and provider number on the claim. Non-physician practitioners, specifically nurse practitioners (NPs), physicians assistants (PAs), clinical nurse specialists (CNSs), and certified nurse midwives (CNMs), can bill their services as incident to services and bill for any level of office visit they provide. Other staff members, such as nurses and medical assistants, can bill their services as incident to, but they are restricted to use of the lowest-established patient E/M office visit code of 99211.

Practices can bill services incident to the care of an NPP, too. For example, say, an NPP treats a patient for hypertension and wants the patient to return to the office for a blood pressure check. The nurse or the medical assistant takes the blood pressure and documents the service. Assuming all other incident to rules are satisfied (e.g., the NPP is in the office suite and immediately available), this service can be billed using the NPP's provider number.

The critical difference between billing incident to a physician and incident to an NPP is the amount reimbursed by Medicare. When you bill incident to a physician, the payment is 100% of the physician fee schedule. When you bill incident to an NPP, you are reimbursed at 85% of the physician fee schedule.

Remember, the employee must be an expense to the practice. CMS allows this expense through employment, leasing, or contracting, but a practice cannot bill incident to services when provided by someone who does not meet these criteria.

Physician Must Initiate Plan of Care.

The physician must see the patient and initiate a plan of care for any other services to be billed incident to. Prior to billing any service as incident to, the physician must see the patient personally. These services must be an integral part of the physician's plan and should be documented in the medical record. An NPP (PA, NP, CNM, CNS) cannot bill a new problem or new patient as incident to the physician. Bill these under the NPP's own provider number.

Many practices are confused by this rule and incorrectly interpret it to mean that an NPP cannot see new Medicare patients. An NPP can see new patients, but you must bill these encounters under the NPP's provider number, not under the physician's provider number.

Here are some examples of a physician-initiated plan of care, carried out by a staff member, and billed incident to (again, assuming all incident to rules are met):

- A physician sees a patient, finds that the patient's blood pressure is slightly elevated, and asks the patient to return to the office every week for a blood pressure check prior to a follow-up visit in six weeks. The medical assistant takes the patient's blood pressure weekly, records it in the chart with a note about how the patient is doing, and the physician sees the patient in six weeks. The blood pressure checks by the medical assistant are billed under the physician's name and provider number, as if the physician had personally provided the service. The blood pressure checks by the medical assistant would be billed as a 99211, as if the physician had provided the service.
- A physician follows a large group of chronically ill patients and shares the care of this group of patients with an NPP. The physician sees and evaluates each patient for initial services in the office. The NPP sees the patients in follow-up every other visit and the physician remains involved in each patient's care. The NPP can bill for the level of service provided and documented as incident to, using the physician name and provider number. This allows the practice to collect 100% of the physician fee schedule.

Direct Supervision Must be Provided.

The physician must supervise the employee providing the incident to services. This does not mean that the physician needs to be in the room while the service is being provided, but must be on-site and immediately available. CMS has clarified this explicitly in its manual:

Direct supervision in the office setting does not mean that the physician must be present in the same room with his or her aide. However, the physician must be present in the office suite and immediately available to provide assistance and direction throughout the time the aide is performing services

Some physicians have tried to stretch the definition of immediately available to include in the hospital attached to the medical office building or in the car and available by phone. But the rule is clear that the physician *must be within the suite of offices*, physically available to provide assistance or direction.

Physician Must Remain Involved with the Patient's Care.

The Medicare manual gives this guidance about the requirement that the physician stay actively involved in the plan of care:

. . . there must be subsequent services by the physician of a frequency that reflects his or her continuing active participation in and management of the course of treatment.

What constitutes "continuing active participation in and management of the course of treatment"? This is not defined in the Medicare manual. There are no clear requirements, but here are some examples that seem perfectly reasonable:

- The physician sees the patient every second or third visit.
- The physician and the NPP meet, review the treatment plan and the patient's present condition and response to treatment, and note that discussion in the medical record. Periodically, the physician sees the patient.
- The physician reviews the notes, comments, and signs off on the plan. Periodically, the physician sees the patient.

Signatures Are Not Required.

There is no requirement that the physician sign a note in which the service is provided by a staff member and the service is billed incident to. In the above examples, some practices may use that method to show that the physician is reviewing the treatment of the patient and staying involved, but Medicare does not require a physician signature. The physician signature on the chart does not "prove" that the physician was in the office and directly supervised the service when it was rendered. If Medicare wants to check if the physician was in the office, it would typically use the appointment schedule.

Clinics and Group Practices

Sometimes, the physician who initiated the plan of care may not be in the office, but another physician is in the office and available to supervise incident to services. In this case, Medicare permits you to bill under the supervising, on-site physician's name and provider number, if you choose incident to billing.

Location

Incident to services must be provided in the physician office or patient's home. Incident to services are not billable in the outpatient department, hospital, nursing home, or other locations.

Welcome to Medicare and Annual Wellness Visits

NPPs may perform the Welcome to Medicare Visit and the Annual Wellness Visits but these should not be billed incident to under the physician's NPI. These visits have their own benefit category and should be billed under the NPP's own NPI number. They will be reimbursed at 85% of the physician fee schedule amount.

Shared Visits

Just when you understood incident to billing, CMS gave us shared visits. Here's what the *Medicare Claims Processing Manual* says about these visits:

Hospital Inpatient/Outpatient/Emergency Department Setting

When a hospital inpatient/hospital outpatient or emergency department E/M is shared between a physician and an NPP from the same group practice and the physician provides any face-to-face portion of the E/M encounter with the patient, the service may be billed under either the physician's or the NPP's UPIN/PIN number. However, if there was no face-to-face encounter between the patient and the physician (e.g., even if the physician participated in the service by only reviewing the patient's medical record) then the service may only be billed under the NPP's UPIN/PIN. Payment will be made at the appropriate physician fee schedule rate based on the UPIN/PIN entered on the claim.

That is, an NPP and a physician can each provide part of an E/M service in the inpatient hospital or outpatient hospital department and bill for the service under the physician's provider number. There are no specific guidelines about what part of these visits need to be performed by the NPP or the physician, or what components need to be documented by each, but here are some general recommendations and requirements:

- The physician must have a face-to-face service with the patient on that day.
- The physician should document the portion of the history, exam, or medical decision making that is clinically relevant. That is, the physician must have a meaningful clinical encounter with the patient and document it.
- The physician encounter can occur before, during, or after the NPP encounter with the patient.
- The service can be billed under the physician's provider number. Combine the level of documentation from the NPP and physician to select the level of service to bill.
- The NPP and physician must be in the same billing group.
- A split/shared service may not be billing in a nursing facility.

Can shared visits be billed in the office? Yes, but only if the incident to requirements are met. That is, if the NPP was seeing the patient for an incident to service, and the physician also saw the patient on the same day, you could bill the service under the physician's provider number. Remember, new patients are never incident to. If the incident to requirements are not met, bill under the NPP's provider number.

Recently, I reviewed some shared visit notes in which the physician had simply countersigned the NPP note. One wrote, "Seen and agree." This type of documentation does not meet the requirements for shared visits. The physician must personally perform a clinically significant portion of the visit and must personally document her participation in the E/M service. In the absence of that service and documentation, bill the service under the NPP provider number. "Seen and agree" or a countersignature can be added to a note at any time and does not document when the physician added the notation or the physician participation in the plan of care.

Here's a summary of shared services rules:

The physician must have a face-to-face service with the patient. The physician should document this by describing a clinically relevant portion of the history and exam performed that day. Which aspects of the history or exam are clinically relevant will vary from patient to patient, but there should be evidence that the visit was more than a social call or "meet and greet" visit.

General supervision is not sufficient. General supervision is not sufficient to bill a shared visit. That is, if the physician did not personally provide a service but simply supervised the work of the NPP, bill the service under the NPP provider number.

Assessment and plan should be noted. The physician should write a sentence about the assessment or plan that adds, clarifies, or supports the NPP's assessment and plan. If the physician sees the patient prior to the NPP note, this sentence or sentences may serve as a recommendation for the NPP work.

The physician should reference the NPP note.

WHY DOES THE OIG CARE?

Incident to services were back on the Office of Inspector General (OIG) Work Plan in 2013.

It's not the first time they've been there. They were on the Work Plan in 2002, 2003, 2004, 2007, and 2008. The fact that it appears year after year tells us a few things. First, incident to billing represents considerable money to the federal government. Second, widespread confusion about the topic persists in physician offices, and Medicare and the OIG know this. Third, to bill correctly every time, a practice needs good systems in place. All of these factors represent opportunity for error, and the OIG knows it.

The 15% differential payment for incident to services matters to CMS.

In August 2009, the OIG released a report about billing for incident to services. (*Prevalence and Qualifications of Non-physician Who Performed Medicare Physician Services*, OEI-09-06-00430). They examined claims submitted by physicians at an unusually high volume in a single day—greater than 24 hours of work. The OIG assumed, correctly, that other healthcare personnel were performing the services and submitting the claims under the physician's provider number. They found that when the total billings exceeded those that could be performed by a physician in one day, more than half of the services were performed by someone else.

The shocking part of the report: unqualified non-physician staff performed 21% of the services that physicians did not personally perform. The executive summary of the report said "In the first 3 months of 2007, Medicare allowed $12.6 million for approximately 210,000 services performed by unqualified non-physicians. These non-physicians did not possess the necessary licenses or certifications, had no verifiable credentials, or lacked the training to perform the service." Some of them were invasive procedures, some were E/M services. They included diagnostic ophthalmology, PT services, cardiac, and diagnostic radiology services.

The message: Don't be creative about what you ask staff to do or train them to do. Be clear about each staff member's scope of practice. There are many services that only a physician, a non-physician practitioner, or other licensed professional can do.

RED FLAGS

There's no substitute for doing a self-audit of your incident to services. Some practices may wonder what level of priority that should be. Here are some red flags and warning signs that, if you spot, should encourage you to start an audit sooner rather than later:

- You don't have a written procedure concerning when to bill your NPPs directly (using their own provider numbers) and when to bill incident to using the physician's name and provider number.
- You always bill your NPPs using the physician's name and provider number.
- You have new staff, either in billing or charge entry.
- You have new NPPs on staff.
- You haven't done an in-service on incident to billing in the last two years.
- NPPs and staff took and failed the quiz at the end of this chapter.
- You're not sure what fields your computer system picks up when assigning a provider number to a claim. Check and see what provider number is picked up for both paper and electronic claims.

COMPLIANCE SOLUTIONS

If your audit of incident to services finds that you are consistently billing these services incorrectly, you have several actions to take. The first is to consult your attorney. Remember, you are required to return to Medicare any funds that you were paid to which you were not entitled.

Second, educate your providers and staff. Have everyone take the self-test at the end of the chapter and make sure that incorrect answers are explained to each person. An educational session for providers, billers, and charge entry staff is critical to ensuring correct billing. Document these activities to prove your efforts at compliance.

In a small office where there is no full-time physician coverage, make sure your appointment schedulers understand that they should schedule nurse visits for Medicare patients when the physician is in the office. Whenever possible, established patients who are being seen incident to a physician's plan of care should be scheduled when a supervising physician is available. Providers may need to indicate this on their encounter forms to alert schedulers to that issue.

Some practices have thrown up their hands and now bill all their NPP services under the NPP's provider number. This certainly simplifies the process, but the practice will not receive as much reimbursement as it otherwise would. Some practices have the NPP indicate on the encounter form whether the care provided was incident to or not. It is preferable to have the NPP indicate this for every encounter.

The NPP would then have one of two choices to circle:

1. This is incident to care (bill under the physician name and provider number).
2. This is not incident to care (bill under my own provider number).

INCIDENT TO TEST

1. You can always bill your NP/PA charges under the MD's provider number, as long as the MD countersigns the note later.	☐ True	○ False
2. The physician must be in the office to bill PA/NP services as incident to, and bill under the MD provider number.	☐ True	○ False
3. NPs and PAs cannot see new Medicare patients.	☐ True	○ False
4. Incident to services are paid at 85% of the physician fee schedule.	☐ True	○ False
5. The physician must stay involved in the plan of care to bill ongoing services by the non-physician practitioner as incident to.	☐ True	○ False

QUIZ ANSWERS

1. You can always bill your NP/PA charges under the MD's provider number, as long as the MD countersigns the note later.

   FALSE. The signature does not prove that the physician was in the office at the time the service was provided. You can bill your NP/PA under the physician provider number only if the service meets all of the requirements of incident to billing.

2. The physician must be in the office to bill PA/NP services as incident to, and bill under the MD provider number.

   TRUE. The physician must be in the suite of offices and available to directly supervise the NP/PA/staff who is providing incident to services.

3. NPs and PAs cannot see new Medicare patients.
   FALSE. NPs and PAs **can** see new Medicare patients, but must bill these encounters under their own provider numbers. New patients cannot be billed as incident to services. Because the patient is new to the practice, the service cannot be part of a physician's plan of care. Bill these visits under the NP/PA provider number or the provider number of the practitioner performing the service.

4. Incident to services are paid at 85% of the physician fee schedule.

   FALSE. But this is a little bit of a trick question. Incident to services tied to the physician's provider number are paid at 100% of the physician fee schedule. However, you can bill incident to a non-physician practitioner. In this case, the incident to service would be paid at 85% of the physician fee schedule.

5. The physician must stay involved in the plan of care to bill ongoing services by the non-physician practitioner as incident to.
   TRUE.

COMPLIANCE PLAN AUDIT SHEET

Auditor Name:	Date of Audit:
Organization Name:	

Incident to Audit Sheet for Non-physician Practitioner Services
Established Patient Visits 99211–99215
For Medicare Patients

To perform this audit, you will need:
- The medical record for each visit
- Access to the appointment schedule for that day
- A copy of the CMS-1500 submitted

Select 10 patients seen by the NPP and billed under the physician provider number. Complete this form for each patient.

Patient ID:	NPP ID:	Physician ID:
Date of Service:	Auditor ID:	Date of Audit:

Answer yes or no to the following questions by checking the appropriate box/circle:

1. Is the patient an established patient?	☐ Yes	◯ No
2. Was this day's service part of a physician-generated plan of care?	☐ Yes	◯ No
3. Was the service performed in the physician's office?	☐ Yes	◯ No
4. Was the staff member who performed the service an employee of the physician or physician practice, a contractor of the physician, or an employee or contractor of the same group that employs the physician?	☐ Yes	◯ No
5. Is the physician remaining involved in the patient's care?	☐ Yes	◯ No
6. Was a supervising physician in the office at the time the service was provided?	☐ Yes	◯ No
7. Did you submit the claim using the provider number of the supervising physician who was in the office?	☐ Yes	◯ No

---

You must answer YES to each of the questions above to bill the service as incident to using the physician name/provider number.

If you answer NO to any one question, bill the service under the PA/NP's provider number.

COMPLIANCE PLAN AUDIT SHEET

Auditor Name:	Date of Audit:
Organization Name:	

Audit Sheet for Non-physician Practitioner Services **New Patients: 99201–99205** **For Medicare Patients**		
To perform this audit, you will need: • The medical record for each visit • A copy of the CMS-1500 submitted Select 5 new patients seen by the NPP. Complete this form for each patient.		
Patient ID:	NPP ID:	Physician ID: (if relevant)
Date of Service:	Auditor ID:	Date of Audit:

Answer yes or no to the following questions by checking the appropriate box/circle:

1. Did the NPP document a new patient visit?	❑ Yes	○ No
2. Is the visit billed under the NPP's provider number?	❑ Yes	○ No

The answer to both questions should be YES.

New patients should be billed under the NPP provider number, not the physician's provider number.

COMPLIANCE PLAN AUDIT SHEET

Auditor Name:	Date of Audit:
Organization Name:	

Incident to Audit Sheet for Nurse Visits Services
Nurse Visits: 99211
For Medicare Patients

To perform this audit, you will need:
- The medical record for each visit
- Access to the appointment schedule for that day
- A copy of the CMS-1500 submitted

Select 10 patients seen by the nurse/medical assistant and billed under the MD provider number. Complete this form for each patient.

Patient ID:	NPP ID:	Physician ID:
Date of Service:	Auditor ID:	Date of Audit:

Answer yes or no to the following questions by checking the appropriate box/circle:

1. Is the patient an established patient?	❒ Yes	◯ No
2. Was this day's service part of a physician-generated plan of care?	❒ Yes	◯ No
3. Was the service performed in the physician's office?	❒ Yes	◯ No
4. Was the staff member who performed the service an employee of the physician, a contractor of the physician, or an employee or contractor of the same group that employs the physician?	❒ Yes	◯ No
5. Is the physician remaining involved in the patient's care?	❒ Yes	◯ No
6. Was the treating physician or a supervising physician in the office at the time the service was provided?	❒ Yes	◯ No
7. Did you submit the claim using the provider number of the supervising physician who was in the office?	❒ Yes	◯ No

You must answer YES to each of the questions above to bill the service as incident to, using the physician name/provider number.

If you answer NO to any one question, you cannot bill the nurse visit.

COMPLIANCE PLAN AUDIT SHEET

Auditor Name:	Date of Audit:
Organization Name:	

Shared Visit Audit Sheet		

To perform this audit, you will need:
- The medical record for each visit
- A copy of the CMS-1500 submitted

Select 10 patients seen by the NPP and MD on the same day and billed under the MD provider number. Complete this form for each patient.

Patient ID:	NPP ID:	Physician ID:
Date of Service:	Auditor ID:	Date of Audit:

You must answer YES to the questions below to bill a shared visit.		
1. Was the service performed in the hospital (inpatient, outpatient, or ED)?	☐ Yes	◯ No
2. Are the Physician and the NPP part of the same group practice?	☐ Yes	◯ No
3. Did both the physician and the NPP have a face-to-face service with the patient?	☐ Yes	◯ No
4. Did the physician document a clinically relevant portion of the E/M service as evidenced by history, exam or MDM?	☐ Yes	◯ No
5. Is the physician entry dated on the date of service for which the shared visit is billed?	☐ Yes	◯ No
6. Is the physician note tied to the NPP note?	☐ Yes	◯ No
Do not bill for only countersignatures or statements that say only "seen and agree."		

CHAPTER 9

Use of Modifier 25

A sk three different physicians to describe the correct use of modifier 25, and you are likely to get three different answers. Even coders can use the modifier inconsistently and incorrectly, causing their carrier to scrutinize their claims. Some insurance companies routinely have ignored modifier 25, refusing to consider the modifier's effect when adjudicating claims. Some insurances require modifier 25 on Evaluation and Management (E/M) services when billed with an immunization or diagnostic test, which is not correct coding. This modifier has a history on the Office of Inspector General (OIG) Work Plan from years past, and was currently on the 2012 Work Plan as part of a review of the use of E/M modifiers during the global period. Like incident to billing discussed in the previous chapter, this issue recurs in the OIG Work Plan. It was frequently a RAC and payer target, as well.

Evaluation and Management Services: Use of Modifiers During the Global Surgery Period (New)

We will review the appropriateness of the use of certain claims modifier codes during the global surgery period and determine whether Medicare payments for claims with modifiers used during the global surgery period were in accordance with Medicare requirements. Prior OIG work has shown that improper use of modifiers during the global surgery period resulted in inappropriate payments. The global surgery payment includes a surgical service and related preoperative and postoperative E/M services provided during the global surgery period. (CMS's *Medicare Claims Processing Manual*, Pub. 100–04, ch. 12, § 40.1.) Guidance for the use of modifiers for global surgeries is in CMS's *Medicare Claims Processing Manual*, Pub. 100–04, ch. 12, § 30. (OAS; W–00–12–35607; various reviews; *expected* issue date: FY 2012; new start)

In 2005, the OIG released a report about the use of modifier 25. It found a high error rate in claims submitted using the modifier; there were a significant number of claims in which there was no separate, significantly identifiable service documented. And, there were claims in which the modifier was used when it was not required. The OIG found that 35% of the claims were incorrectly paid, resulting in $538 million of overpayments. The OIG instructed carriers to increase their education and surveillance of the use of modifier 25. If your carrier is increasing its surveillance, you should review your coding.

Using modifiers is like playing Monopoly™. Use modifiers correctly and it's like landing on Free Parking—your claim sails through the claims processing system and you're paid for multiple services on the first submission. Use modifiers incorrectly and it is like picking the Go to Jail card from the Chance pile. Not only can you not pass Go and collect $200, but your claim is denied and must be resubmitted. If the error was intentionally in your favor, you could face a significant compliance risk.

What is modifier 25 and why is it considered such a source of potential abuse?

Modifier 25 is a CPT® modifier.

> **Modifier 25, Significant Separately Identifiable Evaluation and Management Service by the Same Physician on the Same Day of the Procedure or Other Service:** *It may be necessary to indicate that on the day a procedure or service identified by a CPT® code was performed, the patient's condition required a significant, separately identifiable E/M service above and beyond the other service provided or beyond the usual preoperative and postoperative care associated with the procedure that was performed. A significant, separately identifiable E/M service is defined or substantiated by documentation that satisfies the relevant criteria for the respective E/M service to be reported (see **Evaluation and Management Services Guidelines** for instructions on determining the level of service.) The E/M service may be prompted by the symptom or condition for which the procedure and/or service was provided. As such, different diagnoses are not required for reporting of the E/M service on the same date. This circumstance may be reported by adding modifier 25 to the appropriate level of E/M service.* **Note:** *This modifier is not used to report an E/M service that resulted in a decision to perform surgery. See modifier 57. For significant, separately identifiable non-E/M service, see modifier 59.*

Here are the key points from this definition and other citations:
- Modifier 25 is put on the E/M service, never on the procedure code.
- The diagnosis for the E/M service can be the same as or different from the one for which the procedure was performed.

- The E/M service performed and billed must be separate and significant enough to warrant billing for it, beyond the procedure's normal pre-operative and post-operative work. Per the NCCI edits, the definition of a minor surgical procedure always includes the evaluation of the site, informed consent, the procedure, and post-op instructions for follow up. An E/M service billed on the same day must be above and beyond the usual pre- and post-op work. The *Medicare Claims Processing Manual* says this:

Minor Surgeries and Endoscopies

Visits by the same physician on the same day as a minor surgery or endoscopy are included in the payment for the procedure, unless a significant, separately identifiable service is also performed.

- It is unnecessary to put a modifier on an E/M service when lab or x-ray services are the only other services provided, per CPT® rules. Some payers may have edits that require it.
- Use modifier 25 on the E/M service performed on the same day as the procedure, when the global days for the procedure are 0 or 10 days.
- If the global period for the procedure was 90 days and during the E/M service the physician decided surgery was needed, append modifier 57 to the E/M code.

A High Threshold for Billing Both

According to Medicare policy, payment for procedures includes the pre- and post-work for an E/M service, so has a high threshold for billing both.

Chapter 3 of the *NCCI Manual* says this about billing for a procedure and an E/M service on the same day:

If a procedure has a global period of 000 or 010 days, it is defined as a minor surgical procedure. E&M services on the same date of service as the minor surgical procedure are included in the payment for the procedure. The decision to perform a minor surgical procedure is included in the payment for the minor surgical procedure and should not be reported separately as an E&M service. However, a significant and separately identifiable E&M service unrelated to the decision to perform the minor surgical procedure is separately reportable with modifier 25. The E&M service and minor surgical procedure do not require different diagnoses. If a minor surgical procedure is performed on a new patient, the same rules for reporting E&M services apply. The fact that the patient is "new" to the provider is not sufficient alone to justify reporting an E&M service on the same date of service as a minor surgical procedure. NCCI does contain some edits based on these principles, but the Medicare Carriers have separate edits. Neither the NCCI nor Carriers have all possible edits based on these principles.

And, according to the *Medicare Claims Processing Manual* (100-04) Section 40.1 (B) Services not included in the global surgical package: These services may be paid for separately:

*The initial consultation or evaluation of the problem by the surgeon to determine the need for surgery. Please note that this policy only applies to major surgical procedures. **The initial evaluation is always included in the allowance for a minor surgical procedure;***

New Patient and Procedures

The rules for a new patient and a procedure done on the same day are no different than for established patients; however for a new patient it is more likely that the E/M service will be substantiated. For example, a patient presents to the Emergency Department coughing up blood, and the pulmonary physician is called. After an evaluation, the physician performs a bronchoscopy. Both the E/M service and the bronchoscopy are separately reportable. However, a patient presents with warts, and asked for them to be treated. Report only the wart destruction.

Established Patient and Procedures

Some established patient E/M services are correctly and appropriately billed with a procedure on the same day. A patient may present with new onset shoulder and knee pain. The physician will evaluate the patient's condition; document a medically necessary history, exam, and medical decision making; and bill for the office visit. Then, if the physician decides to inject the patient's knee, she can bill for the E/M service, the knee injection, and the medication. If the physician schedules the patient for a return visit for a re-injection, he or she would bill only for the re-injection at the return visit, in the absence of new problems or symptoms.

The extent of the history, exam, and medical decision making are important factors in billing for an E/M service. For example, a patient calls the office to ask for an appointment for removal of skin tags. The patient presents, the skin tags are removed, and the physician bills for skin tag removal. No E/M service is documented or provided beyond the procedure's typical pre- and post-work. Contrast this with a patient who presents for evaluation of dysfunctional uterine bleeding. The GYN physician takes a history, performs an exam, and decides to obtain an endometrial biopsy that day. Both are separately reportable. A third example is the patient who presents with a suspicious lesion, is evaluated, and scheduled for lesion removal. Sometimes, the physician's schedule does not allow for the procedure to be performed the day the patient presents. In that case, bill for the E/M service on the day of the evaluation, and bill only for the procedure on the day the patient returns.

Planned, repeat, and scheduled procedures are less likely than non-scheduled procedures to require an E/M service with the procedure. An example of this is wound care. Many Wound Care Clinics around the country care for patients who have non-healing wounds, perhaps as a result of chronic disease. At the first visit, the physician will probably bill a new patient or consult visit, along with any necessary debridement. At return visits, he should bill only the medically necessary, documented services. Many of these visits may require debridement only. During some visits, a new lesion may be assessed, an infection may be detected, or the patient's symptoms may have deteriorated and an E/M service is required. In that case, if documented, both services can be billed.

For example, a patient with chronic venous insufficiency, diabetes, and non-healing wounds is seen weekly for wound check and debridement. During the visit in which the wounds are healing and the physician debrides the wound, bill only for the debridement. Contrast that with a return visit at which the patient's condition is worsening. The patient arrives complaining of fever and swelling, and the wound is noted to be larger. The physician opts to culture the wound and treat the patient with antibiotics. Bill for both the debridement and the E/M service.

An unusually high percentage of E/M visits billed with modifier 25 will increase your likelihood of an audit from your payer. Use caution. Don't assume that the physician is entitled to a low-level E/M service with every procedure, or that billing only a low-level service will allow you to fly under the radar. Physicians who always bill a low-level E/M service with every procedure will hear from their payers. Use caution with services such as routine foot care, which are planned in advance. An E/M service is not required for a planned, repeat procedure. Always billing an E/M service with a procedure increases the likelihood of an audit.

Many commercial payers are reviewing notes with modifier 25 at an increased frequency. Medicare Contractors review the percentage of claims submitted with modifier 25 and if there is a significant variance from the norm, will ask for documentation before paying the claim.

Avoid "Always" and "Never"

This is a billing situation that cannot be approached with "always" and "never" statements and policies, such as "We always bill an office visit with every allergy injection"; "All of our patients who have a procedure performed are automatically billed for an office visit or consult"; or "We never bill an E/M service with a procedure." The first two statements are compliance red flags and the last is a revenue issue. Bill for E/M services with procedures when they are reasonable, medically necessary, provided, and documented appropriately.

As we set up our coding, billing, and collection procedures, we strive for uniformity and consistency. We want to "bill everyone the same" and reduce variation in the entire revenue cycle. But, in some situations, it is wise to avoid "always" and "never" statements.

Documentation

The documentation for the E/M service done on the same day as a procedure must meet all of the requirements for the service level billed. For repeat E/M services with procedures, it is more likely to be considered medically necessary when a change occurs in the patient's medical history, exam, or treatment plan. Notes that simply re-state the history and plan do not meet the requirement for an E/M service on the same day as a procedure. Be sure to document the patient's complaints, conditions, and symptoms that are related or unrelated to the problem for which the procedure is performed. The documentation for the E/M service should stand on its own. Do not bill for an E/M service when the documentation mainly describes the procedure.

Colonoscopy

Medicare considers the pre-op E/M work for a screening colonoscopy to be part of the procedure, so do not bill for an E/M service prior to the procedure. It's incorrect to bill an E/M service on the same day as a colonoscopy with a modifier 25. The Centers for Medicare & Medicaid Services (CMS) has repeatedly clarified that it will not pay for a pre-op evaluation for a *screening* colonoscopy. Pre-operative evaluations for *diagnostic* colonoscopies are payable.

WHY THE OIG CARES

Using modifiers bypasses the claims editing systems that CMS has instructed carriers to implement in their claims adjudication systems. This allows the provider to be paid automatically, without review of the documentation. The Office of Inspector General (OIG) study finds that modifier 25 was applied in far more situations than was warranted by the payment rules.

In the *Medicare Claims Processing Manual* section about the global periods, carriers are instructed that they do not need to routinely review claims with a modifier 25, but should in the following case:

> *When carriers have conducted a specific medical review process and determined, after reviewing the data, that an individual or group have high statistics in terms of the use of modifier "25," have done a case-by-case review of the records to verify that the use of modifier "25" was inappropriate, and have educated the individual or group as to the proper use of this modifier.*

Your own billing pattern will determine whether your claims submitted with modifier 25 receive scrutiny.

RED FLAGS

Beware of policies that result in "always" and "never" situations. If you "always" bill an E/M service with every procedure or you "never" do so, you risk 1) using the modifier incorrectly and out of compliance with definitions and rules or 2) losing revenue. If you can, run a report by provider to see how often the practice uses the modifier. Check your denial reports to see if you are receiving denials for the modifier. Pay particular attention to high-level E/M services with minor procedures and established patients with procedures. List the procedures your practice performs frequently and determine whether these procedures are performed on a scheduled, repeat basis. The billing and documentation for those services deserves particular attention.

COMPLIANCE SOLUTIONS

The solutions to problems you find in using modifier 25 depend on the work process you have for assigning modifiers to claims. Significant variation exists among practices in how modifiers are selected. In some practices, the physician is responsible for selecting and adding all modifiers to the charging document. In some practices, if the practitioner indicates that both a procedure and an office visit were performed, the biller or coder automatically adds the modifier to the E/M service at the time of charge entry. In the most conservative practices, all notes are reviewed before the modifier is appended to the office visit.

This, of course, is a highly compliant procedure but has the disadvantage of being expensive and causing delays in submitting claims.

The process you use should depend on whether your audit shows you are attaching modifier 25 when the documentation does not support it; not billing for services that are medically necessary, provided, and documented; or billing correctly. In the first two cases, education of providers and billing staff is recommended.

Excessive or Incorrect Use of Modifier 25

If your audit reveals that you are billing for E/M services on the same day of a procedure that are not medically necessary, provided, or documented, review notes before submitting claims until the problem is solved. Ask a member of your billing or coding staff to review the documentation prior to submitting the claims. Educate all staff members and, in particular, any providers whose audit results indicate frequent errors. Allow the providers to indicate the use of the modifier without review only when your coding staff is satisfied that the service meets the requirements.

If you find that your office is submitting claims with the modifier on the code for the procedure instead of the E/M service, educate your charge entry staff! Review denial reports to make sure you are resubmitting denied claims and not losing reimbursement. Remember, if you find that you have collected money to which you were not entitled, you are required by law to return it to government payers. Consult your healthcare attorney.

Services Provided But Not Billed

Physicians, non-physician practitioners, and coders are often so interested in compliance and so afraid of breaking rules that they do not bill for services that are medically necessary, provided, and documented. Sometimes, a single payer's policy is misunderstood to be the rule for everyone. Physicians remember that a staff member told them that they could not bill for an E/M service with a procedure and that they should have the patient come back for the procedure. The actual communication is that a certain payer has a policy about that, but the understanding is that it is a more generally applicable rule when it isn't.

The most effective solution to this fear of billing non-compliantly is education with citations. Show the providers and coders the regulations as outlined in the CPT® book, the *Medicare Claims Processing Manual* and carrier instructions. Providers complain that the rules change from year to year and different coders tell them different things. This is true. But although some payers have used varying reimbursement policies in years past for recognizing or not recognizing modifier 25, the rules have been in place for many years.

COMPLIANCE PLAN AUDIT SHEET

Auditor Name:		Date of Audit:
Organization Name:		

Use of Modifier 25

To perform this audit, you will need:
• The medical record for each visit
• Access to the patient account

Select 10 patients who have had a procedure and an E/M service performed. Complete this form for each patient.

Modifier 25 is used to indicate that a procedure was performed on the same day as a significant, separately identifiable E/M service. Append the modifier to the E/M service. All services billed must be **medically necessary**. Whether or not to bill the E/M service with a modifier requires some judgment. This audit sheet will help you assess these claims consistently and correctly.

Patient ID:		Physician or NPP ID:	
Date of Service:	Auditor ID:		Date of Audit:

To bill an office visit with a procedure you must answer YES to the following six questions:		
Is an office visit documented?	☐ Yes	○ No
Is a procedure documented?	☐ Yes	○ No
Does the procedure have a 0 or 10-day global period?	☐ Yes	○ No
For the office visit:		
Is there a history documented?	☐ Yes	○ No
For a *new patient*, is a separate exam documented?	☐ Yes	○ No
Is there an assessment/plan noted in the chart?	☐ Yes	○ No
Feel more confident if the answer to either of these two questions is YES:		
Was this the first time the physician saw the patient for this problem?	☐ Yes	○ No
Was a second problem addressed during the office visit?	☐ Yes	○ No
Show caution about billing for both if the following is true:		
Is the procedure a repeat procedure?	☐ Yes	○ No
Do not bill if the answer to either of these questions is YES:		
Did the patient return to the office solely to have the procedure done because the physician did not have time to do the procedure on the day of the diagnosis?	☐ Yes	○ No
Does the note seem to be all re-cap of a previously taken history and plan?	☐ Yes	○ No
Was the minor surgical procedure provided for an obvious, clear problem, such as treatment for warts or simple laceration repair?	☐ Yes	○ No

CHAPTER 10

Billing for E/M Services During the Global Period

I n 2012, the Office of Inspector General (OIG) Work Plan included a review of Evaluation and Management (E/M) services during the global period. This is a continuation of work started in 2011. Although this topic is not on the current year's Work Plan, it is a frequent RAC target and private payers will also audit when E/M services are reported during the global period. If we look back, we can see that it was a Work Plan item in 2006, as well. E/M services provided in the global period are a concern for both the OIG and the Centers for Medicare & Medicaid Services (CMS). Most E/M services provided in the global period are not separately reportable, i.e., payable. However, using certain modifiers can override claims editing and allow a medical practice to be paid for E/M services. Also, CMS is interested in whether the relative value units (RVUs) assigned to surgical procedures reflect the work provided in the post-op period. Here is how the OIG Work Plan describes their current interest:

Evaluation and Management Services During Global Surgery Periods

We will review industry practices related to the number of E&M services provided by physicians and reimbursed as part of the global surgery fee. CMS's Medicare Claims Processing Manual, Pub. No. 100-04, ch. 12, § 40, contains the criteria for the global surgery policy. Under the global surgery fee concept, physicians bill a single fee for all of their services that are usually associated with a surgical procedure and related E&M services provided during the global surgery period. We will determine whether industry practices related to the number of E&M services provided during the global surgery period have changed since the global surgery fee concept was developed in 1992. (OAS; W-00-09-35207; various reviews; expected issue date: FY 2011; work in progress)

To understand how to audit and review these services for yourself, it is important to understand the definition of the global surgical package. Once the global surgical package is defined, this chapter will discuss what E/M services are included in the package and when a surgical group can bill for other E/M services. The correct use of modifiers is critical in billing and being paid for E/M services during the global period, both at the start of the package and after the procedure itself.

Selected Modifier Definitions for Use in the Global Period

The modifiers that are important during the global period are described in full in Appendix A of the CPT® book. Here are their brief descriptions:

- **Modifier 24**: Unrelated Evaluation and Management Service by the Same Physician During a Postoperative Period
- **Modifier 25**: Significant, Separately Identifiable Evaluation and Management Service by the Same Physician on the Same Day of the Procedure or Other Service
- **Modifier 54**: Surgical Care Only
- **Modifier 55**: Postoperative Management Only
- **Modifier 56**: Preoperative Management Only
- **Modifier 57**: Decision for Surgery

CMS Definition of the Global Period

The section about the global package in the *Medicare Claims Processing Manual* is lengthy and detailed. It can be found in its entirety by downloading Chapter 12 of the *Medicare Claims Processing Manual* (http://www.cms.gov/Regulations-and-Guidance/Guidance/Manuals/Internet-Only-Manuals-IOMs.html). Publication 100-04, and looking at Section 40.

CPT® procedure codes covered by the global concept are identified in the Medicare Physician Fee Schedule Data Base by an entry in Field 16 with 000, 010, and 090. ZZZ are surgical add-on codes. There is no post-op work associated with these, because the post-op work is associated with the primary procedure. Codes with the indicator YYY in Field 16 allow the contractor to determine the global period, which will be 0, 10, or 90 days.

Payment for surgical procedures includes all of the components described in the surgical global package. From the *Medicare Claims Processing Manual*:

> The Medicare approved amount for these procedures includes payment for the following services related to the surgery when furnished by the physician who performs the surgery. The services included in the global surgical package may be furnished in any setting, e.g., in hospitals, ASCs, physicians' offices. Visits to a patient in an intensive care or critical care unit are also included if made by the surgeon. However, critical care services (99291 and 99292) are payable separately in some situations.

Preoperative Visits—Preoperative visits after the decision is made to operate beginning with the day before the day of surgery for major procedures and the day of surgery for minor procedures;

Intra-operative Services—Intra-operative services that are normally a usual and necessary part of a surgical procedure;

Complications Following Surgery—All additional medical or surgical services required of the surgeon during the postoperative period of the surgery because of complications which do not require additional trips to the operating room;

Postoperative Visits—Follow-up visits during the postoperative period of the surgery that are related to recovery from the surgery;

Postsurgical Pain Management—By the surgeon;

Supplies—Except for those identified as exclusions; and

Miscellaneous Services—Items such as dressing changes; local incisional care; removal of operative pack; removal of cutaneous sutures and staples, lines, wires, tubes, drains, casts, and splints; insertion, irrigation and removal of urinary catheters, routine peripheral intravenous lines, nasogastric and rectal tubes; and changes and removal of tracheostomy tubes.

When provided by the surgeon, the services listed above are not separately reportable. The payment for them is included in the global payment for the surgery. If an E/M service is provided within the global period and meets the requirements for modifiers 24, 25, or 57, the service may be separately reported.

CMS's definition of follow-up care includes all medical or surgical follow-up unless a return trip to the operating room is required. Complications, wound infections, pain control problems—all of these visits and procedures done in the office are part of the global payment per Medicare. CPT® describes the follow-up care as "typical" follow up and allows for billing of complications. It can be difficult to keep track of the two sets of payment rules in an office.

Separate Payment for E/M Services

According to the *Medicare Claims Processing Manual*, these services are not included in the global package:

Services Not Included in the Global Surgical Package

Contractors do not include the services listed below in the payment amount for a procedure with the appropriate indicator in Field 16 of the MFSDB. These services may be paid for separately.

- *The initial consultation or evaluation of the problem by the surgeon to determine the need for surgery. Please note that this policy only applies to major surgical procedures. The initial evaluation is always included in the allowance for a minor surgical procedure;*
- *Services of other physicians except where the surgeon and the other physician(s) agree on the transfer of care. This agreement may be in the form of a letter or an annotation in the discharge summary, hospital record, or ASC record;*
- *Visits unrelated to the diagnosis for which the surgical procedure is performed, unless the visits occur due to complications of the surgery;*
- *Treatment for the underlying condition or an added course of treatment which is not part of normal recovery from surgery;*
- *Diagnostic tests and procedures, including diagnostic radiological procedures;*
- *Clearly distinct surgical procedures during the postoperative period which are not re-operations or treatment for complications. (A new postoperative period begins with the subsequent procedure.) This includes procedures done in two or more parts for which the decision to stage the procedure is made prospectively or at the time of the first procedure. Examples of this are procedures to diagnose and treat epilepsy (codes 61533, 61534-61536, 61539, 61541, and 61543), which may be performed in succession within 90 days of each other;*
- *Treatment for postoperative complications which requires a return trip to the operating room (OR). An OR for this purpose is defined as a place of service specifically equipped and staffed for the sole purpose of performing procedures. The term includes a cardiac catheterization suite, a laser suite, and an endoscopy suite. It does not include a patient's room, a minor treatment room, a recovery room, or an intensive care unit (unless the patient's condition was so critical there would be insufficient time for transportation to an OR);*
- *If a less extensive procedure fails, and a more extensive procedure is required, the second procedure is payable separately;*
- *For certain services performed in a physician's office, separate payment can no longer be made for a surgical tray (code A4550). This code is now a Status B and is no longer a separately payable service on or after January 1, 2002. However, splints and casting supplies are payable separately under the reasonable charge payment methodology;*
- *Immunosuppressive therapy for organ transplants; and*

- *Critical care services (codes 99291 and 99292) unrelated to the surgery where a seriously injured or burned patient is critically ill and requires constant attendance of the physician.*

Separate payment can be made for the initial evaluation for a major surgical procedure done at any time in relation to the surgery. For minor procedures, the service must meet the criteria for use of modifier 25.

E/M Services Provided with Minor Procedures and Endoscopy

See the chapter on the Use of Modifier 25 for more detailed discussion of this topic. In brief, an E/M service is payable on the same day as a minor procedure *only* when the E/M service is a significant, separately identifiable, medically necessary service. An example of this would be the care for a new patient or consultation on the same day as a bronchoscopy. It would not be required for a scheduled repeat procedure at which no other issues were addressed.

The payment for a minor surgical procedure always includes the pre-operative assessment of the site, obtaining consent, the procedure, and instructions for aftercare.

Decision for Surgery

The E/M visit at which the decision to perform a major surgery is made is always separately payable, even if provided the day of or the day before the surgery. A surgeon who provides any E/M service (consult, hospital service, ED visit, or office visit) and makes the decision at this visit to perform a procedure with a 90-day global period may be paid for that service. If the visit at which the decision for surgery is made is done two days prior to the surgery or before, no modifier is needed. If the E/M service results in the decision for surgery the same day or the next day, use modifier 57 on the E/M service.

Hospital-Mandated History and Physical Exam

It is common for a physician to see a patient for an initial evaluation, schedule surgery at a mutually convenient time, and then need to see the patient back for a hospital-mandated history and physical (H&P). Often, this H&P is dictated in the hospital system for a service done in the office. This is not a separately reportable service, per both CPT® and CMS. These services will often be paid if submitted to the payer, because they appear as an established patient visit with a covered diagnosis code. This was a query addressed in the May 2009 volume of *The CPT® Assistant*. Asked if this H&P was a separately reportable service, *The CPT® Assistant* responded with this: "*If the surgeon sees a patient and makes a decision for surgery and then the patient returns for a visit where the intent of the visit is the preoperative H&P, and this service occurs in the interval between the decision-making visit and the day of surgery, regardless of when the visit occurs (1 day, 3 days, or 2 weeks), the visit is not separately billable as it is included in the surgical package.*"

Begins and Ends

The global period for minor surgical procedures or endoscopies starts the day of the procedure. These are services with a 0 or 10-day global period. Procedures with 0 global days include only the care provided that day. Procedures with 10 global days include follow up for 10 days. Count the day after the procedure as day one. The global period for a major surgical procedure, one with a 90-day period, starts the day before the procedure. Count 90 days starting the day after the procedure to determine the end of the global period. CMS is making changes to the global period starting in 2017. In 2017, services that now have a 10 day global period will have no global period. In 2018, services that now have a 90 day global period will have no global period.

Complications in the Post-Op Period

The CPT® definition of the global package varies from Medicare's definitions. The CPT® definition allows physicians to bill post-op complications during the global period. CMS does not. According to CMS, only complications requiring a return trip to the OR are separately payable in the post-op period. Bill for return trips to the OR with the 78 modifier. These, of course, are procedures and not E/M services.

For commercial carriers that follow CPT® rules, complications during the global period are separately reportable. Bill an E/M service with modifier 24 and use the complication as the diagnosis. Practices should check with their commercial payers to see if they recognize the use of modifier 24 for this situation.

Unrelated E/M Services During the Post-Op Period

A physician who performs a procedure may bill and be paid for an *unrelated* E/M service during the post-op period if the E/M service is unrelated to the surgery. The documentation for these services should support that the service was unrelated to the surgery. Submit a diagnosis code that indicates the reason for the visit. For example, an Orthopedic surgeon may treat a patient's knee with a surgery that has a 90-day global period. During the post-op period, the patient returns to the surgeon for treatment of carpal tunnel syndrome. This is a separately reimbursable service. Bill the E/M service with a modifier 24 and a diagnosis for an unrelated problem.

Critical Care Services

Critical care services (99291 and 99292) are payable before or after a surgical procedure if the surgeon is providing care unrelated to the surgery. The *Medicare Claims Processing Manual* gives two examples of this. One is for the care of a critically ill or burned patient who needs critical care unrelated to the surgical procedure. The patient must be critically ill and require the constant attendant of the physician.

The second example, according to the *Claims Processing Manual*, is if the critical care is "above and beyond, and, in most instances, unrelated to the specific anatomic injury or general surgical procedure performed." These would be "potentially unstable" patients or ones who suffer from conditions that pose significant threats to their life or health. Report 99291 and 99292 with modifier 25 or modifier 24 (for post-op care). Document that the critical care was unrelated and report an appropriate ICD-9 code [e.g., 800.0–959.9 (except 930–939)].

Document time in the medical record. Do not include time spent in performing the surgical procedures or other codes bundled into critical care. See the chapter on critical care in this book. These claims may require prepayment contractor review. In many instances, there is an intensivist or hospitalist who is managing the nonsurgical related care. In that case, the surgeon would not report critical care in the postop period.

Post-Op by Another Physician

A surgeon who is covering for another surgeon and provides post-op care does not separately report the service, whether or not the surgeons are in the same group. This is true whether the care is provided in the office or hospital.

Hospitalists often provide care in the post-op period for hospitalized patients. The CMS manual notes that care by other physicians is separately reportable. However, use caution. The surgeon is paid to manage the post-op care of the patient. This includes input/output, fluids, nutrition, bowel movements, wound care, pain management, ambulation, rehabilitation plans, and discharge planning and management. A medicine physician should only bill for medically necessary problems, and should provide care only as long as is medically necessary. For example, a frail elderly patient is admitted for a hip fracture, but has multiple underlying problems including coronary artery disease, hypertension, and chronic kidney disease. It is medically necessary for a medicine physician to address and manage those problems while the patient is in the hospital. No one would expect the Orthopedist to write the orders for Lasix or to manage stage IV chronic kidney failure. But other patients may be entirely stable in the post-op period and would not require any or daily visits by an Internist or Family Physician. Those physicians should sign off of the care of the patient when all of the issues are related to post-op management.

Global Package Provided by Different Surgeons

There are times when one surgeon provides the surgical service and another provides the post-op care. This might occur if a patient has a major surgical procedure while traveling and returns home for the post-op care. In this case, the surgeon who performs the procedure and the surgeon who provides follow-up care both report the same date of service and procedure code. The operating surgeon uses modifier 54 on the claim for the surgical care and the physician who provides the post-op care uses modifier 55. The date on which the care was assumed must be indicated on the claim form by the surgeon providing the post-op care. The surgeon providing the post-op care may bill only after providing the first post-op service. Both surgeons should keep a written transfer of care in the patient's record.

WHY THE OIG CARES

Using modifiers allows payment for E/M services at the start of the global period, on the day of the procedure, and during the global period. CMS defines the fee for the global surgical package as including all of the E/M services in the period, unless the services meet the criteria for separate payment described in the previous section of this chapter. CMS does not want to pay twice for the same service or to pay separately for services included in the global package.

CMS pays physicians for surgical procedures using the global surgical fee concept. This includes payment for the procedure and "related E/M services during global surgical period," according to the OIG Work Plan. This warns physicians not to bill and contractors not to pay separately for E/M services provided in the global package.

RED FLAGS

Always and Never

Warning bells go off in my head when I hear statements like this:

- "We always bill an office visit with a procedure."
- "We never bill an office visit with a procedure."
- "The H&P is always part of the global. We've never billed for it. Ever."
- "I ran a report, and we don't have any services billed with a 25, 57, or 24 modifier."

If your practice performs procedures in the office or the hospital, be concerned if:

- You never submit claims with the modifiers identified at the start of this chapter: 24, 25, 54, 55, 56, 57;
- You have denials based on the use of these;
- There is no written policy for assigning these modifiers;
- Physicians do not know what is included in the global package;
- Your practice does not have a quick, easy reference that indicates the global days;
- No one in the office understands the surgical global indicators in the Medicare Physician Fee Schedule Data Base; or
- Your coders always assign modifiers without reviewing the documentation.

COMPLIANCE SOLUTIONS

Buy or download a copy of the Medicare Physician Fee Schedule Data Base and review the surgical indicators, global period, and facility versus non-facility RVUs for the services you perform. It is a large Excel file. There are coding programs and books for purchase that provide the information in a more manageable form.

It is important for surgical practices to send a coder, and if possible, a physician, to specialty training. Many commercial vendors and specialty societies offer terrific, specialty-specific resources. I know I run the risk of sounding like a broken record, but although you can find codes by searching your CPT® and ICD-9 books, understanding the coding and reimbursement rules requires time and effort.

Review your denials for claims submitted with the modifiers listed in this chapter. Run a report that shows your use of these modifiers and review your process for assigning these modifiers. Who is responsible: the physician? The coder? If the coder assigns the modifier, does the coder review all or a sampling of the documentation?

If your surgical practice provides emergency surgery to patients who do not live in your area, are you using modifiers 54 and 55 correctly, breaking up the surgical package? It would be incorrect to bill the surgical procedure without a modifier—globally—if the practice only provided the surgery. Similarly, if your practice provides the follow-up for the surgical care, it's incorrect to bill these with E/M services. These should be billed with modifier 55.

COMPLIANCE PLAN AUDIT SHEET

Auditor Name:	Date of Audit:
Organization Name:	

Use of Modifier 57		

To perform this audit, you will need:
- The medical record for each visit
- Access to the patient account

Select 10 patients who had a major surgical procedure performed the same day or the day after the surgeon first saw the patient for that condition.

Patient ID:	Physician ID:	Date of Procedure:
Date of E/M Service:	Auditor ID:	Date of Audit:

You must answer YES to all of these questions to bill for an E/M services, a 57 modifier, and be paid for that service on the same day or the day after surgery:

1. Does the procedure have a 90-global day period?	❏ Yes	◯ No
2. Was an E/M service performed on the same day or the day before the procedure?	❏ Yes	◯ No
3. Does the documentation show that the decision for surgery was made at this visit?	❏ Yes	◯ No

Note: It is a CMS rule that modifier 57 is used on surgical procedures with a 90-global day period, not a CPT® rule.

COMPLIANCE PLAN AUDIT SHEET

Auditor Name:	Date of Audit:
Organization Name:	

Use of Modifier 24 **This is an audit sheet for Medicare.**

To perform this audit, you will need:
- The medical record for each visit
- Access to the patient account

Remember, CPT®'s definition of follow-up in a global period is different from Medicare's.

Patient ID:	Physician ID:	Date of Procedure:
Date of E/M Service:	Auditor ID:	Date of Audit:

You must answer YES to all of the questions below.

1. Identify procedures billed with a 24 modifier. Circle the global period for that service: 10 days 90 days Was this E/M service billed after a procedure during the global period?	☐ Yes	○ No
2. Was the reason for the visit unrelated to the surgery?	☐ Yes	○ No
3. Were the symptoms described unrelated to the surgery?	☐ Yes	○ No
4. Was the assessment and diagnosis for a problem different than the surgery?	☐ Yes	○ No
5. Was a different diagnosis used?	☐ Yes	○ No

COMPLIANCE PLAN AUDIT SHEET

Auditor Name:	Date of Audit:
Organization Name:	

Use of Modifier 54 and 55		
To perform this audit, you will need: • The medical record for each visit • Access to the patient account Identify 10 patients for whom the practice provided a surgical service for which the patient's ZIP Code/state of home residence was far away from the practice locale.		
Patient ID:	Physician ID:	Date of Procedure:
Date of E/M Service:	Auditor ID:	Date of Audit:

Billed with no modifier:		
If you billed the service with no modifier, did you provide the pre-op, surgical care, and post-op care?	❑ Yes	○ No
If yes, this is correct. If you did not provide the post-op care, resubmit the claim with a modifier 54, surgical care only.		
Billed with modifier 54:		
If you billed the service with modifier 54, did you provide only the surgical care?	❑ Yes	○ No
If yes, this is correct. Your medical record should show that the surgical service was provided by another surgeon.		

CHAPTER 11

Initial Preventive Physical Examinations and Annual Wellness Visits

The Medicare Modernization Act passed in July 2004 provided new Medicare beneficiaries with a once-in-a-lifetime benefit: The Welcome to Medicare visit, also known as the Initial Preventive Physical Examination (IPPE). Medical practices can bill and be paid for this preventive service. It is not a typical, preventive medicine exam, as defined by CPT® codes 99381–99397. Those visits remain non-covered services. The goal of the IPPE as defined by the benefit, is two-fold: 1) health promotion and disease detection and 2) education, counseling, and referral for other Medicare-covered preventive benefits. In developing the definition of the service and the required components, CMS relied heavily on recommendations from the U.S. Preventive Services Task Force (USPSTF), clinical medical societies, and comments from physicians and others in the healthcare field. No existing CPT® code described the set of services that are required for the IPPE, so CMS developed a set of temporary HCPCS codes to use to bill for the services.

In 2011, CMS developed a benefit called an Annual Wellness Visit (AWV). The AWV is defined as an initial or subsequent wellness visit, and shared some characteristics with the IPPE. This chapter will describe both the Welcome to Medicare visit and the initial and subsequent Annual Wellness Visits, and provide audit sheets for both.

IPPE: What Medicare Beneficiary Is Eligible?

Only beneficiaries who enroll in Medicare on or after January 1, 2005 are eligible for an IPPE service and they are eligible only for 12 months from the date of their enrollment. This is a one-time benefit, meaning Medicare will pay for this only once for a beneficiary—and only within the first 12 months of the beneficiary's enrollment. Most beneficiaries become eligible for Medicare at age 65, and so are eligible for the benefit between ages 65 and 66. However, some beneficiaries with end-stage renal disease or other disability may become eligible for Medicare at a younger age. They are eligible for this benefit during the first year in which they are enrolled in Medicare, which may not necessarily coincide with age 65.

Physicians, PAs, NPs and CNSs Can Provide IPPE

Physicians and qualified non-physician practitioners (NPPs) can provide the service. The Medicare definition of physicians includes Medical Doctors, Doctors of Dental Surgery, Doctors of Podiatric Medicine, Doctors of Optometry, and Chiropractors. However, physicians and practitioners must practice within their scope of practice, so practically speaking, only MDs and DOs are qualified to perform the service.

Physician Assistants, Nurse Practitioners, and Clinical Nurse Specialists can bill for the service, also within their own state scope of practice, but Clinical Nurse Midwives may not provide and bill for the service. Submit the service under the National Provider Identifier (NPI) of the clinician who provides the service. The service may not be billed incident to a physician service. Do not bill for this service provided by an NPP under the physician's provider number.

Components of the IPPE

The Initial Preventive Physical Exam (IPPE) requires each of these components:
1. History
   - Review of the individual's medical and social history with particular attention to modifiable risk factors for disease;
   - Past medical history, surgical history, including experience with illnesses, hospital stays, operations, injuries, allergies, and treatment;
   - Current medications and supplements, including calcium and vitamins;
   - Family history, including a review of medical events in the patient's family, including diseases that may be hereditary or place the individual at risk; and
   - Social history, including history of alcohol, tobacco, and illicit drug use; diet; and physical activities.
2. Review of individual's potential for depression
   - Review of the individual's potential for depression, including current or past experiences with depression or other mood

disorders based on the use of an appropriate screening instrument for persons without a current diagnosis.

3. Review of the patient's functional ability and level of safety
   - Review of the individual's functional ability and level of safety based on the use of appropriate screening questions or a screening questionnaire, including hearing impairment, activities of daily living, falls risk, and home safety.

4. Physical exam to include the following
   - An examination to include height, weight, blood pressure, calculation of body mass index, a visual acuity screen, and other factors as deemed appropriate by the MD or NPP based on the patient's history and current clinical standards.

5. Performance and interpretation of an EKG if needed (Optional)
   - Initially, performance and interpretation of an EKG was required as part of the visit; however, this is now optional.

6. Education, counseling, and referral, as appropriate, based on the results of the first five elements.

7. With patient consent, discussion of end-of-life issues.

8. Education, counseling, and referral, including a brief ***written plan given to the patient*** (such as a checklist) recommending the appropriate screening and other preventive services covered by Medicare. Include these items in the plan:
   - Pneumococcal, influenza, and hepatitis B vaccines and their administration;
   - Screening mammography;
   - Screening pap smear and screening pelvic exams ;
   - Prostate cancer screening services;
   - Colorectal cancer screening tests;
   - Diabetes outpatient self-management training services;
   - Bone mass measurements;
   - Screening for glaucoma;
   - Medical nutrition therapy services for individuals with diabetes or renal disease;
   - Cardiovascular screening blood tests;
   - Diabetes screening tests; and
   - Screening test for abdominal aortic aneurysm when ordered as part of the IPPE for patients who meet the criteria of needing the screening.

Not Your Typical Preventive Medicine Service

There are some real differences between the IPPE as defined by CMS and a typical "annual exam." Obtaining the patient's medical, social, and family history is fairly standard. However, notice that there is no specific requirement for the extent of the review of systems for this service, and the required exam is extremely limited.

There are two very specific screening requirements in the visit, not formally included in many annual exams: 1) The patient *must* be screened for depression using a standard, industry-acceptable test for use in patients without a known diagnosis of depression; and 2) screening questions must be asked to assess the patient's safety, hearing, and functional ability at home.

The required physical exam is brief: height, weight, calculation of body mass index, blood pressure, visual acuity, and whatever other physical exam elements the provider deems appropriate based on the patient's history and screening results. An EKG and interpretation became optional in 2009, and discussion of end-of-life issues, with the patient's consent, was added as an optional component. Finally, the physician or NPP must provide counseling on the first five elements and provide counseling and a *written plan* to the patient in regards to obtaining other covered Medicare Part B screening services (those listed in #8 above).

Co-pays and Deductibles

The co-pay and deductible are waived for the IPPE. The optional EKG, however, is subject to co-pay and deductible.

Diabetes Screening

The Medicare Modernization Act also added a diabetes screening benefit for beneficiaries who meet certain requirements at specific intervals. Not all beneficiaries are eligible for this benefit—only those who meet the screening criteria.

- Testing furnished to an individual at risk for diabetes
- Benefit paid using existing CPT® codes per the lab fee schedule
- **82947**: Glucose; quantitative, blood (except reagent strip)
- **82950**: Post glucose dose (includes glucose)
- **82951**: Glucose: tolerance test (GTT) three specimens, includes glucose

- Requires ICD-9 code V77.1, special screening for diabetes mellitus

Covered yearly for beneficiaries with these health risks:
- Hypertension
- Dyslipidemia
- Obesity, defined as a body mass index greater than or equal to 30kg/m2
- Previous identification of an elevated impaired fasting glucose
- Previous identification of impaired glucose tolerance
- A risk factor consisting of two of the following:
  - Overweight, defined as a body mass index greater than 25kg/m2, but less than 20
  - A family history of diabetes
  - A history of gestational diabetes mellitus or delivery of a baby weighing greater than 9 lbs.
  - 65 years of age or older

For patients with pre-diabetes, two screening tests per 12-month period are covered. Pre-diabetes is defined as:
- Previous fasting glucose level of 100-125 mg/dL, or
- A 2-hour post-glucose challenge of 140-199 mg/dL

For individuals previously diagnosed with diabetes, no screening coverage is provided because these tests are covered for diagnostic, medically indicated reasons.

Cardiovascular Screening

The MMA provides for cardiovascular screening blood tests for the early detection of cardiovascular disease or abnormalities associated with an elevated risk for that disease. This coverage is provided once every five years and requires specific diagnosis codes. The covered tests are total cholesterol, HDL-cholesterol, and triglycerides. The CPT® codes are 80061 (lipid profile), 82465 (cholesterol), 83718 (lipoprotein), and 84478 (trigylcerides).

These tests can be ordered as a lipid panel or individually, limited to one of each individual test or a combination every five years. The laboratory should use a lab Advance Beneficiary Notice (ABN) if it believes the patient may have had the test more frequently than once in the past five years. The ABN notifies the patient that Medicare may not cover the screening test due to frequency limitations. Without an ABN, the patient is not financially responsible. These services are paid under the lab fee schedule, using CPT® codes.

Payment for the cardiovascular screening tests requires the use of specific diagnosis codes:

V81.0 Special screening for cardiovascular, respiratory, and genitourinary diseases, ischemic heart disease

V81.1 Special screening for cardiovascular, respiratory, and genitourinary diseases, hypertension

V81.2 Special screening for cardiovascular, respiratory, and genitourinary diseases, other and unspecified cardiovascular conditions

This benefit is for screening, for individuals not already diagnosed. Patients with high cholesterol or lipids may have these lab tests performed diagnostically, with a covered ICD-9 code as is medically necessary.

Screening for Abdominal Aortic Aneurysm

Beginning in 2007, Medicare began paying for ultrasound screening for abdominal aortic aneurysm (AAA) if it is recommended to eligible patients during the Welcome to Medicare visit. Males between the ages of 65 and 75 who have a family history of AAA, or who have smoked more than 100 cigarettes in their lifetimes, and for whom Medicare has never paid for a screening for AAA before, are eligible for the screening. At that time, only patients referred as a result of the Welcome to Medicare visit are eligible. Now, however, CMS will pay for one screening for eligible patients, even if they are not referred at the IPPE. The diagnostic facility would bill with HCPCS code G0389.

Advance Beneficiary Notice

Do you need an ABN when you provide the IPPE? Sometimes yes, sometimes no. What if the patient had an IPPE at the office of another doctor and you are providing a second IPPE to a beneficiary? Because a second IPPE is never covered by Medicare, no ABN is required. Some beneficiaries routinely receive medical care near a summer and a winter home, so getting two IPPEs can occur. However, the physician may bill the patient in this instance without obtaining an ABN.

What if you are providing the service outside of the 12-month period in which Medicare covers the service? Then, yes, you do need to execute an ABN with the patient. The beneficiary is eligible to receive the IPPE only within twelve months of his enrollment date in Medicare. If the doctor has a doubt as to the enrollment date and provides the service, the provider should get an ABN from the patient. Without an ABN in this case, the provider is financially responsible in case of a denial due to lapsing of the statutory time limitation.

HCPCS codes

The relevant Medicare codes for IPPE are:

G0402: Initial Preventive Physical Examination; face-to-face visit services limited to new beneficiary during the first 12 months of Medicare enrollment

G0403: Electrocardiogram, routine ECG with at least 12 leads with interpretation and report, performed as a component of the initial preventive physical exam

G0404: Tracing only, without interpretation and report performed as a component of the initial preventive physical exam

G0405: Interpretation and report performed as a component of the initial preventive physical exam

The screening EKG performed on the same day as the IPPE should be reported with the HCPCS code above. Using the CPT® code 93000 will result in a denial.

Office Visit on the Same Day

Medicare initially proposed that billing an office visit on the same day as the IPPE be limited to a "Level 2" E/M code. However, CMS received numerous comments and removed this restriction. If you provide a medically necessary, separate E/M service, that is, an office visit for an acute or chronic problem, you may bill for that service. Append modifier 25 to the office visit.

CMS states in the November 15, 2005 *Federal Register*, "We do not believe this scenario will be the typical occurrence and, therefore, we will monitor the utilization patterns for the level 4/5 new or established office or other outpatient visits codes being reported with the IPPE" (p. 66290). Physicians should take this warning seriously and make sure they adequately document the key components of the office visit that they bill with the IPPE.

Other Preventive Medicine Services

Often, clinicians will provide a pelvic and breast exam (G0101) and obtain a pap smear (Q0091) on the same day as the Welcome to Medicare exam. Bill for these separately.

Annual Wellness Visits: Initial and Subsequent

As part of healthcare reform, Medicare now pays for an Annual Wellness Visit (AWV). Hold the champagne—it's not what you or your doctors think of as an annual exam. In fact, it's has more in common with the Welcome to Medicare visit than an annual exam. The CPT® codes for preventive medicine (99381–99397) remain non-covered, routine services. Bill them to Medicare and they will be denied; they are patient due services. The Annual Wellness Visit will be billed to Medicare with new HCPCS codes developed for this purpose.

Like the IPPE, these visits may not be billed incident to a physician's services. If an NPP provides the service, it must be billed under the NPP's NPI number. The visit is paid based on the NPI number of the rendering physician, at 100% of the physician fee schedule for physicians and at 85% of the physician fee schedule for NPPs.

During the first year a patient is enrolled in Medicare, the beneficiary will be eligible only for the Welcome to Medicare visit described above. The Welcome to Medicare visit, or Initial Preventive Physical Exam (IPPE), is a once-in-a-lifetime benefit, billed with HCPCS code G0402.

The Annual Wellness Visits are defined as initial and subsequent. The initial AWV is reported with code G0438 and the subsequent AWV is reported with G0439. These visits do not have new and established patient designations, so a clinician can perform an initial visit on an established patient to the practice. The initial AWV may be performed on patients who have been enrolled in Medicare for more than a year, or one year after the patient had the Welcome to Medicare visit. A patient is eligible for the subsequent wellness visit one year after the initial wellness visit. An example might help sort out eligibility.

Bob is 70 and has been enrolled in Medicare since he was 65. Starting January 1, 2011, Bob is eligible for an Initial Annual Wellness Visit. Let's say he receives that AWV on April 29, 2011. He is eligible for a subsequent wellness visit after 11 full months have passed. Jock, however, became eligible for Medicare on July 1, 2012. He is eligible for the Welcome to Medicare visit until June 30, 2013. Let's say he receives it on May 7, 2012. He is eligible for his initial Annual Wellness Visit one year later, and for a subsequent wellness visit after 11 full months have passed.

What about patients who receive part of their care in the sunny south during the winter (lucky ones) and part of their care in the north during the summer? Can they receive the visits twice, once in the summer and once in the winter, since they are cared for by two different physicians? No, these visits are per beneficiary, not per physician.

What is required during the initial Annual Wellness Visit?

- Have patient complete a Health Risk Assessment.
- Establish/update the patient's past medical, family, and social history.
- List the patient's current medical providers, suppliers, and all medications, including supplements.
- Record height, weight, calculated BMI, BP, and "other routine measurements."
- Review potential for depression using an appropriate screening tool.
- Review individual's functional level of safety and ability to perform activities of daily living, fall risk, and home safety.
- Detect cognitive impairment via direct observation, discussion, review of medical records, or discussion with family.
- Establish a personalized, written preventive plan for the next 5–10 years with services recommended by the U.S. Preventive Task Force.
- Furnish personalized health advice that includes listing of patient's conditions, risk factors, treatment recommendations, and methods to decrease risk factors such as smoking, obesity, etc.

Health Risk Assessment

As part of the initial and subsequent AWV, the patient must complete a Health Risk Assessment (HRA). CMS did not provide a template or form to use for the HRA, but the Centers for Disease Control and Prevention (CDC) has a framework for one in a document entitled, "A Framework for Patient-Centered Health Risk Assessments." Some specialty societies have provided templates for their members. The HRA is intended to be completed by the patient prior to the visit, and includes questions regarding health behaviors, lifestyle, exercise, diet, and smoking. The clinician reviews the HRA and includes the information in the personalized plan and recommendations given to the patient.

Co-pay and Deductible

The co-pay and deductible are waived.

Other Services That Can Be Provided on the Day of the AWV

A physician or NPP may bill for other services provided on the same day as the AWV. A patient could receive the pelvic and breast exam, for example, on the day of the AWV. Any other preventive services that are covered by Medicare can be provided on the same day as the wellness visit.

A separate E/M service may also be billed on the day of a wellness visit; however, no part of the documentation used for the wellness visit may be used to determine the level of service for the E/M. The *Medicare Claims Processing Manual* states, *"Some of the components of a medically necessary E/M service (e.g., a portion of history or physical exam portion) may have been part of the IPPE or AWV and should not be included when determining the most appropriate level of E/M service to be billed for the medically necessary, separately identifiable, E/M service."*

When thinking about the Annual Wellness Visit, consider what other healthcare team members could perform part of the service. In an Open Door Forum in February 2011, CMS confirmed that a staff member could perform part of the service. This could include taking the history and screening required for the visit and doing some of the health education.

WHY DOES THE OIG CARE?

The IPPE made its appearance in the fee schedule in 2005. A year later, it appeared on the Office of Inspector General (OIG) Work Plan and was included in the 2007 Work Plan as a work in progress. These changes in coverage represent a huge new cost to the Medicare program. According to the Federal Register, providing the IPPE cost the program $40 million in 2005. The cholesterol and lipid screening cost $50 million and the diabetes screening $20 million in 2005. With an investment like this, contractors, CMS, and the OIG will all be interested in the accuracy of billing for the new service.

Both the IPPE and the AWV have a specific list of services that must be provided and documented for the practice to report the service. Know that some of the services are not typically provided during a preventive medicine exam, such as depression screening and the written plan for screening services.

Physician practices that do not take the time to read the fine print may find that their typical preventive medicine service does not qualify for payment under the definition of these wellness visits. Some practices may try to use preventive medicine forms or electronic health record templates that they already have in place. This service will require significant changes in both the provision of service and the record keeping that goes with the service.

A physician group that decides not to provide the IPPE or the Annual Wellness Exam may have complaints from patients who expect the service as part of their Medicare benefits.

RED FLAGS

Many practices have gotten off to a slow start in providing this new benefit to Medicare patients. Some physicians do not know what the components of the service are and may try to use the HCPCS codes when the components are not documented. Here are some warning signals about providing the IPPE and the AWV:

- You do not have new forms or templates set up to provide the service;
- Your billing office has received patient complaints about the provision of the service;
- You do not have a copy of a written plan for each patient for whom you have provided the service;
- You don't have a way to monitor beneficiary eligibility and don't know if you are scheduling the patient for a typical physical exam, the IPPE, or the AWV;
- You don't have templates built into your EMR for each of these services; or
- Your billing office receives multiple complaints from patients who were expecting one of these wellness visits but were billed for a different service.

COMPLIANCE SOLUTIONS

If you have not had a formal training session to explain this new service to physicians, NPPs, schedulers, coders, and billers, do so immediately. Add this topic to your next provider or staff meetings.

If you find that your providers are using previously existing preventive medicine forms or electronic health record templates, you should worry that you are not meeting all of the criteria for the new code.

If you are not giving patients a written plan for screening tests when they leave the office after receiving their IPPE or a written 5–10 year plan at the time of the AWV, you are not providing the service as described and should not bill for it.

Use the audit sheet below as a guide to check if the paper form or electronic health record has all of the required components.

COMPLIANCE PLAN AUDIT SHEET

Auditor Name:	Date of Audit:
Organization Name:	

Initial Preventive Physical Examination			
For this audit you will need the medical record for a specific encounter and the chart. Select 10 patients per provider who have an encounter billed at any location. Complete this form for each encounter. For procedural and ICD-9-CM auditing, use other sheets in this book.			
Patient ID:		Provider ID:	
Auditor ID:	Date of Audit:	DOS:	
For every service billed with G0402, answer these questions. You must answer YES to all of the questions (except question 6 in some cases) to bill G0402:			
1. Does the medical history include past medical and surgical history, including experience with illnesses, hospital stays, operations, allergies, injuries, and treatment?	☐ Yes	◯ No	
Does the medical history include current medications and supplements, including calcium and vitamins?	☐ Yes	◯ No	
Does the note document family history, including a review of the medical events in the patient's family, including diseases that may be hereditary or place the individual at risk?	☐ Yes	◯ No	
Does the social history contain information about alcohol, tobacco, illicit drug use, diet, and physical activities?	☐ Yes	◯ No	
2. Is there a depression screening instrument completed for the visit?	☐ Yes	◯ No	
3. Are the patient's functional ability and level of safety evaluated (includes review of hearing impairment, activities of daily living, falls risk, and home safety)?	☐ Yes	◯ No	
4. Does the exam document BP, height, weight, calculation of body mass index, and a test for visual acuity?	☐ Yes	◯ No	
5. Was a screening EKG performed at the time of the visit and the results reviewed with the patient? (This is optional as of January 1, 2009.)	☐ Yes	◯ No	
6. If appropriate, did the physician counsel the patient about issues uncovered in the history and exam and refer the patient?	☐ Yes	◯ No	

7. Did the physician provide a written plan to the patient reminding the patient that he or she is eligible for and is being referred for other Medicare covered Part B screening services? *These covered Part B screening services include:* • *Pneumococcal, influenza, and hepatitis B vaccines and their administration* • *Screening mammography* • *Screening pap smear and screening pelvic exams* • *Prostate cancer screening services* • *Colorectal cancer screening tests* • *Diabetes outpatient self-management training services* • *Bone mass measurements* • *Screening for glaucoma* • *Medical nutrition therapy services for individuals with diabetes or renal disease* • *Cardiovascular screening blood tests* • *Diabetes screening tests*	❑ Yes	⭘ No
8. For services provided after January 1, 2009, did the physician discuss end-of-life issues with the patient or document that the patient declined to discuss these?	❑ Yes	⭘ No

AUDIT SHEET FOR THE AWV, INITIAL OR SUBSEQUENT

Annual Wellness Visit		
Patient ID:		Provider ID:
Auditor ID:	Date of Audit:	DOS:

For every service billed with G0438 or G0439, answer these questions. You must answer YES to all of the questions to bill G0438 or G0439. G0439 is an update.

1. Does the medical history include past medical and surgical history, including experience with illnesses, hospital stays, operations, allergies, injuries, and treatment?	☐ Yes	○ No
Does the medical history include current medications and supplements, including calcium and vitamins?	☐ Yes	○ No
Does the note document family history, including a review of the medical events in the patient's family, including diseases that may be hereditary or place the individual at risk?	☐ Yes	○ No
Does the social history contain information about alcohol, tobacco, illicit drug use, diet, and physical activities?	☐ Yes	○ No
2. Is there a depression screening instrument completed for the visit?	☐ Yes	○ No
3. Are the patient's functional ability and level of safety evaluated (includes review of hearing impairment, activities of daily living, falls risk, and home safety)?	☐ Yes	○ No
4. Does the exam document BP, height, weight, calculation of body mass index? (Waist circumference may be used instead of BMI.)	☐ Yes	○ No
5. Is there a health risk assessment?	☐ Yes	○ No
6. Did the clinician assess cognitive impairment, if any?	☐ Yes	○ No
Is there a list of current medical providers and suppliers documented?	☐ Yes	○ No
7. Was personalized advice given, including a list of patient's conditions, risk factors, treatment recommendations, and methods to decrease risk factors given to the patient? This should incorporate HRA information and information obtained in the screenings.	☐ Yes	○ No
8. Is there a personalized, written plan for the next 5–10 years with services recommended by the USPTF documented, and notation that a copy was given to the patient?	☐ Yes	○ No

CHAPTER 12

Teaching Physician Rules

The teaching physician rules are Medicare regulations that govern billing for attending physician services provided jointly with residents in a teaching setting. For the purpose of this chapter, attending physician and teaching physician are used interchangeably. Using the teaching physician rules, the attending physician bills for services provided jointly by a resident and a teaching physician in a graduate medical education (GME) program. These rules have undergone revision and refinement over the years, yet the basics have not changed. However, the specifics about when the teaching physician must be present and who must document the attendance are different for E/M services, services selected based on time, and surgical services. Large hospitals have run afoul of these regulations and paid large settlements to the federal government.

Definitions Are Key

The first section of these rules in the Medicare Claims Processing Manual, entitled *Supervisory Physicians in a Teaching Setting*, is a list of definitions. This chapter of the manual is included on your CD. On the Centers for Medicare & Medicaid Services (CMS) web site, download Chapter 12 of Publication 100-04, Ch. 12, and look at Section 100: http://www.cms.hhs.gov/Manuals/IOM/list.asp.

These definitions are from the CMS manual:

> For purposes of this section, the following definitions apply:
> - ***Resident***—*An individual who participates in an approved graduate medical education (GME) program or a physician who is not in an approved GME program but who is authorized to practice only in a hospital setting. The term includes interns and fellows in GME programs recognized as approved for purposes of direct GME payments made by the FI. Receiving a staff or faculty appointment or participating in a fellowship does not by itself alter the status of "resident." Additionally, this status remains unaffected regardless of whether a hospital includes the physician in its full time equivalency count of residents.*

- **Student**—An individual who participates in an accredited educational program (e.g., a medical school) that is not an approved GME program. A student is never considered to be an intern or a resident. Medicare does not pay for any service furnished by a student. See §100.1.1B for a discussion concerning E/M service documentation performed by students.
- **Teaching Physician**—A physician (other than another resident) who involves residents in the care of his or her patients.
- **Direct Medical and Surgical Services**—Services to individual beneficiaries that are either personally furnished by a physician or furnished by a resident under the supervision of a physician in a teaching hospital making the reasonable cost election for physician services furnished in teaching hospitals. All payments for such services are made by the FI for the hospital.
- **Teaching Hospital**—A hospital engaged in an approved GME residency program in medicine, osteopathy, dentistry, or podiatry.
- **Teaching Setting**—Any provider, hospital-based provider, or nonprovider setting in which Medicare payment for the services of residents is made by the FI under the direct graduate medical education payment methodology or freestanding SNF or HHA in which such payments are made on a reasonable cost basis.
- **Critical or Key Portion**—That part (or parts) of a service that the teaching physician determines is (are) a critical or key portion(s). For purposes of this section, these terms are interchangeable.
- **Documentation**—Notes recorded in the patient's medical records by a resident, and/or teaching physician or others as outlined in the specific situations below regarding the service furnished. Documentation may be dictated and typed or hand-written, or computer-generated and typed or handwritten. Documentation must be dated and include a legible signature or identity. Pursuant to 42 CFR 415.172 (b), documentation must identify, at a minimum, the service furnished, the participation of the teaching physician in providing the service, and whether the teaching physician was physically present.

In the context of an electronic medical record, the term 'macro' means a command in a computer or dictation application that automatically generates predetermined text that is not edited by the user.

When using an electronic medical record, it is acceptable for the teaching physician to use a macro as the required personal documentation if the teaching physician adds it personally in a secured (password protected) system. In addition to the teaching

*physician's macro, either the resident or the teaching physician must
provide customized information that is sufficient to support a medical
necessity determination. The note in the electronic medical record
must sufficiently describe the specific services furnished to the specific
patient on the specific date. It is insufficient documentation if both
the resident and the teaching physician use macros only.*

- ***Physically Present**—The teaching physician is located in the same
room (or partitioned or curtained area, if the room is subdivided to
accommodate multiple patients) as the patient and/or performs a
face-to-face service.*

Surgical Services

The definition of a minor procedure for the purposes of the teaching
physician rules is not the same as the usual definition of a minor
procedure: one with 0 or 10 global days. Here, the definition is a
procedure that takes fewer than five minutes. For minor procedures of
fewer than five minutes, the attending physician must be present for the
entire procedure. The resident may document the attending physician's
presence and the teaching physician can sign the resident's note.

For endoscopy, the attending physician must be present from the
time the scope is introduced until it is withdrawn. "Scope in, scope
out," as the saying goes. Watching the procedure via a monitor is not
sufficient. The resident or operating room nurse may document the
attending physician's presence; the attending can sign the note.

For major surgery, an attending physician must be present for the
key or critical portions of the surgery. The attending physician decides
which portions of each surgery are key or critical. If the attending
physician leaves the operating room she must be available to personally
intervene immediately should that become necessary and should not be
performing another procedure at that time.

If the teaching physician is supervising one major surgery, His or
her presence may be noted in the medical record by the nursing staff
or by the resident physician. There is no requirement that the teaching
physician personally document their attendance for a single major
procedure. For two overlapping surgeries, the attending physician must
be present for the key or critical portions of both surgical procedures
and must be available to provide assistance. The key and critical
portions may not take place at the same time. If the teaching physician
is not immediately available for one of the surgeries, the teaching
physician must designate another physician, not a resident, in his or

her absence or the service is not billable. The teaching physician must personally document his participation in a major surgery and tie that documentation to the resident note.

If a teaching physician is working on three overlapping surgeries, no payment is allowed under the physician fee schedule.

Teaching anesthesiologists who supervise a single anesthesia resident may bill as if they personally provided the service. The teaching anesthesiologist must document in the patient's medical record that she was present during the key or critical portion of the service. If the anesthesiologist is supervising more than one procedure concurrently, this is paid using the medical direction rules. Again, the teaching physician must personally document his participation in the anesthesia and tie his notes to the resident's note.

Teaching Physician Rules for Evaluation and Management Services

The supervision of the provision of Evaluation and Management (E/M) services by residents when billing the services under the teaching physician provider number seems complicated when you read the *Medicare Claims Processing Manual*. There are multiple scenarios and differing requirements based on whether the code requires two of the three key components of history, exam, and medical decision making or all three components to meet the requirements for that code.

However, it is actually quite simple. To bill for E/M services performed jointly by a resident physician and an attending physician under the attending physician's provider number, the attending physician must: 1) personally document that she performed or was present during the performance of an E/M service during the key or critical components and 2) personally document her participation in the clinical care of that patient. The attending physician also ties his or her note to the residence note. If these criteria are met, the organization can use the combination of both of these services to select the level of service. The attending physician note should reference or tie to the resident's note in some way.

Here are examples of acceptable documentation from the CMS manual:

- *Admitting Note: "I performed a history and physical examination of the patient and discussed his management with the resident. I*

> reviewed the resident's note and agree with the documented findings
> and plan of care."

- *Follow-up Visit:* "Hospital Day #3. I saw and evaluated the patient.
  I agree with the findings and the plan of care as documented in the
  resident's note."

- *Follow-up Visit:* "Hospital Day #5. I saw and examined the patient. I
  agree with the resident's note except the heart murmur is louder, so I
  will obtain an echo to evaluate."

- *Initial or Follow-up Visit:* "I was present with the resident during the
  history and exam. I discussed the case with the resident and agree
  with the findings and plan as documented in the resident's note."

- *Follow-up Visit:* "I saw the patient with the resident and agree with
  the resident's findings and plan."

- *Initial or Follow-up Visit:* "I saw and evaluated the patient. Discussed
  with resident and agree with resident's findings and plan as
  documented in the resident's note."

- *Follow-up Visit:* "See resident's note for details. I saw and evaluated
  the patient and agree with the resident's finding and plans as
  written."

- *Follow-up Visit:* "I saw and evaluated the patient. Agree with
  resident's note but lower extremities are weaker, now 3/5; MRI of L/S
  spine today."

These examples clearly show that the attending was physically present,
saw and evaluated the patient, and participated in the clinical care of the
patient. The attending then ties his attestation to the resident's note. A
resident must have written a note, and it helps if the notes are labeled
by specialty, such as "Cardiology resident" and "Cardiology attending."
When multiple sets of physicians round on a patient in a single day, it
can be confusing to know what resident and what attending are working
together without these identifying headings.

Time-Based Codes

For time-based codes, only the time of the attending physician counts.
That is, the time spent by the resident may not be included in the time
used to determine the CPT® code based on time. The attending physician
must personally document in the medical record the amount of time he
spent in the provision of care. Resident time may not be included. These
types of services include some time-based psychotherapy codes, critical

care services, discharge management based on time, prolonged services, care plan oversight, and E/M codes selected based on time.

The resident may not document the attending physician's participation or time. In the case of critical care, the resident's notes may add detail to the care provided, such as the condition of the patient or the treatment, but the attending physician must document the time he spent, the condition of the patient, and the interventions and treatments performed personally. Do not include time spent teaching in the time reported or the resident's time.

For discharge code 99239, only the attending physician's time counts. The attending physician must personally document her participation and the time spent.

For an E/M service billed on the basis of time (because more than 50% of the total time was spent in counseling or coordination of care), the attending physician's time is the only time that counts. The attending physician must personally document the participation and the time and the medical record. If only the attending physician sees the patient, then the attending physician must document his participation solely.

Primary Care Exception Rule

There's an allowance in the teaching physician rules for billing for services under the primary care exception rule. This allows an attending physician to bill for resident services provided in a primary care setting without having a face-to-face service with the patient. To bill for services under the primary care exception, the organization must qualify for this exception and must keep a written record of its qualification. The practice does not need to send this to its contractor or CMS, but must keep it on file within the organization. To qualify, the practice must provide primary care services to patients who consider that practice to be their primary care practice. In general, the resident must follow the same patients over the course of the residency. This rule typically is used by Family Practice, Internal Medicine, and OB/GYN, but can be also Psychiatry in some circumstances.

In billing under the primary care exception rule, the attending physician must be onsite, supervising four or fewer residents at any one time, and can have no other responsibilities than the supervision of these residents during that time. The medical record should show that the attending physician documented in the patient's individual medical record the review and supervision of the resident in the care of the patient. Typically this supervision occurs immediately after the resident physician sees the patient. The attending physician must personally document in the patient's medical record her supervision and involvement in the care.

For the organization to bill using the primary care exception, each resident must have been in a GME program for longer than six months.

There are limited codes that can be billed under the primary care exception. These include 99201–99203, 99211–99213, and the Welcome to Medicare visit, G0402. The Initial Annual Wellness visit and the Subsequent Annual Wellness Visit also may be billed under the primary care exception rules (G0438, G0439).

Modifiers

Bill for attending physician services provided in part by a resident under the teaching physician rules with a GC modifier. If billing for services under the primary care exception rule, use modifier GE. These modifiers do not affect payment.

Medical Students

Tucked into the CMS definitions at the beginning of this chapter was the definition of a student and the statement that "Medicare does not pay for any service furnished by a student." Services performed by any type of student (medical student, NP, PA) are not reportable services. An attending may not co-sign these notes and bill for the service as if the student were a resident. For an E/M service, a student may document what any staff member may document—the review of systems and past medical, family and social history—and an attending may count that documentation in selecting a level of service, if referenced. In practice, a student documents a complete note but it is not used as a basis for billing.

WHY THE OIG CARES

Medicare provides funding for training residents in approved programs and pays the hospital through the Medicare contractor for these services. In addition, services provided jointly between an attending and a resident may be billed to Medicare if the guidelines are followed. The sums of money are large and both CMS and the Office of Inspector General (OIG) intend to protect the Medicare and Medicaid trust funds. Most teaching hospitals and their compliance departments learned from the large paybacks in the past and have developed stringent auditing and compliance activities in this area.

Although the rules have not changed significantly in past years, the variance in the rules based on the type of service being provided has confused physicians. Attending physicians have multiple responsibilities and supervise dozens of residents over the course of a year, and this can be challenging. It is the attending's responsibility, however, to follow these rules. Claims are submitted under the attending's provider number.

RED FLAGS

Students in an organization are always a red flag. There are many practices not defined as teaching practices that periodically have a nurse practitioner student or medical student rotate through the practice. Be sure everyone understands that student services may never be billed for.

Confusion about the use of the teaching physician modifiers is a cause for alarm. The modifiers should not be applied to all services billed by an attending; some of those services are personally provided and not jointly provided with a resident. Apply the modifier only to services provided jointly. It is a good use of compliance time to review the application of the GC and GE modifiers.

If the group has not audited teaching physician services in the past year, that is a red flag. Most compliance departments in teaching hospitals do include the auditing of teaching physician rules as part of their compliance audit. It would be prudent to be sure that is happening.

ACTION ITEMS

Educate, review, and audit. Educating residents is particularly challenging simply from a scheduling perspective. Getting everyone in a room at the same time, awake, is virtually impossible. Many groups find that a series of mandatory educational sessions with the same content provided at varying times over a few days is effective. A 7:00 a.m. meeting, a lunch meeting, a session at 4:00 p.m., all with food, can be effective. Spread these over several days to increase the likelihood that all residents will have the opportunity to attend one session.

CMS also has a very informative and short fact sheet regarding teaching physician rules that all staff and physicians can read quickly: "Guidelines for Teaching Physicians, Interns, and Residents." It is easy to read and understand, and could be included in the orientation of new staff and residents.

Use the audit sheets in this chapter to audit services provided under the teaching physician rules.

COMPLIANCE PLAN AUDIT SHEET

Auditor Name:	Date of Audit:
Organization Name:	

Teaching Physicians Time-Based Codes Audit Sheet			
To perform this audit, you will need: • The medical record for each visit • A copy of the CMS-1500 submitted			
Select 10 patients billed under the attending physician provider number in which a resident participated in the care.			

Patient ID:	Physician ID:	Resident ID:
Date of Service:	Auditor ID:	Date of Audit:

Answer YES to these questions:		
1. Did the attending physician personally document his or her time in the medical record?	☐ Yes	○ No
2. Did the attending physician personally document the participation in the care?	☐ Yes	○ No
3. Does the time documented match the time described for that code in the CPT® book?	☐ Yes	○ No
4. For an E/M service, did the attending physician note his or her own total time, that more than 50% of the visit was spent in counseling, and the nature of the counseling?	☐ Yes	○ No
The next four questions are for <u>critical care services</u>:		
1. Was the patient critically ill?	☐ Yes	○ No
2. Did the attending physician provide a critical care service, such as writing orders, documenting treatment, and status in the progress note and documenting his or her participation?	☐ Yes	○ No
3. Did the attending physician document his or her own time in the medical record, and his or her participation in the care? (The resident note may be used to supplement the attending physician note.)	☐ Yes	○ No
4. Did the practice use modifier GC?	☐ Yes	○ No

COMPLIANCE PLAN AUDIT SHEET

Auditor Name:	Date of Audit:
Organization Name:	

Teaching Physicians Primary Care Exception Audit Sheet		

To perform this audit, you will need:
- The medical record for each visit
- A copy of the CMS-1500 submitted

Select 10 patients billed under the attending physician provider number in which a resident participated in the care.

Patient ID:	Physician ID:	Resident ID:
Date of Service:	Auditor ID:	Date of Audit:

1. For services billed under the primary care exception: Does the organization qualify?	☐ Yes	◯ No
2. Is the attending physician supervising four or fewer residents at a time?	☐ Yes	◯ No
3. Was supervising the residents the only responsibility of the attending physician for that period?	☐ Yes	◯ No
4. Are all of the services billed using only codes 99201–99203 and 99211–99213 or G0402, G0438, G0439?	☐ Yes	◯ No
5. Did the attending physician document in the patient's individual medical record the review and direction of the patient's care?	☐ Yes	◯ No
6. Has the resident been in a GME program for longer than six months?	☐ Yes	◯ No
7. Was modifier GE used?	☐ Yes	◯ No

COMPLIANCE PLAN AUDIT SHEET

Auditor Name:	Date of Audit:
Organization Name:	

Teaching Physicians Surgical Services Audit Sheet—Minor Procedures		
To perform this audit, you will need: • The medical record for each visit • A copy of the CMS-1500 submitted Select 10 patients billed under the attending physician provider number in which a resident participated in the care.		
Patient ID:	Physician ID:	Resident ID:
Date of Service:	Auditor ID:	Date of Audit:

1. Was the attending physician present for the entire minor procedure lasting fewer than five minutes?	☐ Yes	◯ No
2. Is the attending physician presence documented in the medical record by the physician, the resident, or an assisting nurse?	☐ Yes	◯ No
3. Was modifier GC used?	☐ Yes	◯ No

COMPLIANCE PLAN AUDIT SHEET

Auditor Name:	Date of Audit:
Organization Name:	

Teaching Physicians Endoscopy Audit Sheet				
To perform this audit, you will need: • The medical record for each visit • A copy of the CMS-1500 submitted				
Select 10 patients billed under the attending physician provider number in which a resident participated in the care.				
Patient ID:	Physician ID:		Resident ID:	
Date of Service:	Auditor ID:		Date of Audit:	
1. Was the attending physician personally present from the insertion of the scope to the withdrawal of the scope?		☐ Yes		○ No
2. Is the attending physician's presence documented in the medical record by the attending physician, the resident, or the operating nurse?		☐ Yes		○ No
3. Was the service billed with modifier GC?		☐ Yes		○ No

COMPLIANCE PLAN AUDIT SHEET

Auditor Name:	Date of Audit:
Organization Name:	

Teaching Physicians Audit Sheet—Major Surgical Procedures		

To perform this audit, you will need:
- The medical record for each visit
- A copy of the CMS-1500 submitted

Select 10 patients billed under the attending physician provider number in which a resident participated in the care.

Patient ID:	Physician ID:	Resident ID:
Date of Service:	Auditor ID:	Date of Audit:

*For supervision of all **single major procedures**:*

1. For a single major surgical procedure, is the attending physician's care documented in the medical record? (Does not have to be by the attending personally)	☐ Yes	○ No
2. Does this documentation show that the attending physician was in the operating suite for the key or critical portion of this service?	☐ Yes	○ No
3. Was the attending physician immediately available for assistance during any time he or she was not in the operating suite?	☐ Yes	○ No
4. Was the service billed with modifier GC?	☐ Yes	○ No

*For supervision of **overlapping surgeries**:*

1. Was the teaching physician present for the critical or key portions of both? (Only the teaching physician determines which portions of the surgery are key or critical.)	☐ Yes	○ No
2. If the attending physician was not immediately available during portions of one of the surgeries, did the teaching physician transfer responsibility to another teaching physician, not to a resident?	☐ Yes	○ No
3. For two overlapping services, did the attending personally document his/her participation?	☐ Yes	○ No
4. Was the service billed with modifier GC?	☐ Yes	○ No

If the teaching physician supervised more than three overlapping surgeries, the services are not billable.

COMPLIANCE PLAN AUDIT SHEET

Auditor Name:	Date of Audit:
Organization Name:	

Teaching Physicians Audit Sheet E/M Services

To perform this audit, you will need:
- The medical record for each visit
- A copy of the CMS-1500 submitted

Select 10 patients billed under the attending physician provider number in which a resident participated in the care.

Patient ID:	Physician ID:	Resident ID:
Date of Service:	Auditor ID:	Date of Audit:

You must answer YES to all of these questions.

1. Did the attending physician and the resident both have a face-to-face service with the patient?	❏ Yes	○ No
2. Did the attending physician personally document that he or she saw the patient with a statement like one of these: "saw and evaluated," "performed an H&P," "was present with the resident during the history and physical," "saw the patient with the resident"?	❏ Yes	○ No
3. Did the attending physician personally document his or her participation in the clinical care of that patient with statements like these: "I agree with the findings and plan of care as documented in the resident's note," "I agree with the resident's note except that her lungs are wheezy so I will obtain a chest x-ray to evaluate," "I agree with the resident's finding and plan," or " Discussed with residents and agree with residents finding as planned as documented in the resident's note"?	❏ Yes	○ No
4. Does the attending physician's note reference a specific resident by name or specialty for any day that has more than one resident and more than one attending rounding ? (That is, can you tell that a specific attending physician was linking his or her note to a specific resident? This can be done by naming the resident, "Dr. Jones saw this patient" or by naming the specialty of the resident, "the cardiology resident." If the notes are labeled cardiology attending, cardiology resident, you can assume that these notes belong together.)	❏ Yes	○ No
5. Was the service billed with modifier GC?	❏ Yes	○ No

CHAPTER 13

Care Plan Oversight

Some physicians perform the services that describe care plan oversight (CPO) without ever submitting a claim for the service. Others submit claims for CPO without understanding the rules and knowing exactly what patients are eligible and what services are covered. Although CPO has not made an appearance on the OIG Work Plan since 2006, if a practice is providing the service, it is important to understand the requirements and documentation.

Typically, physicians are not paid for talking on the phone and coordinating care between face-to-face Evaluation and Management (E/M) services to their patients. The CPT® book defines telephone services as distinct CPT® codes, but most insurance companies do not pay for these services, and Medicare gives them a status indicator of N for non-covered. However, care plan oversight is one of the few services that Medicare pays that is not a face-to-face service.

There are two services that are defined by the Centers for Medicare & Medicaid Services (CMS) and described using HCPCS codes.

> **G0181**: physician supervision of a patient receiving Medicare-covered services provided by a participating Home Health Agency (patient not present) requiring complex and multidisciplinary care modalities involving regular physician development and/or revision of care plans, review of subsequent reports of patient status, review of laboratory and other studies, communication (including telephone calls) with other health care professionals involved in the patient's care, integration of new information into the medical treatment plan and/or adjustment of medical therapy, within a calendar month, 30 minutes or more.

> **G0182**: physician supervision of a patient receiving Medicare-covered services provided by a participating hospice (patient not present) requiring complex and multidisciplinary care modalities involving regular physician development and/or revision of care plans, review of subsequent reports of patient status, review of laboratory and other studies, communication (including telephone calls) with other health care professionals involved in the patient's

care, integration of new information into the medical treatment plan and/or adjustment of medical therapy, within a calendar month, 30 minutes or more.

The definition and billing requirements of CPO are specific and detailed, and the reimbursement makes learning them worthwhile. The services must be personally performed by the physician or non-physician practitioner (NPP)—not a member of the staff. At least 30 minutes of services defined as CPO must be provided within a calendar month. The time spent, a description of the services, and the date must be included and the physician or NPP must sign the documentation.

In addition, CPO can only be billed by one physician in a single month's time, and it must be the same physician who certified the home health or hospice services. If the CPO is billed by the NPP, the NPP must have a collaborative agreement with the physician who signed the certification for home health or hospice services. The patient must require complex, multidisciplinary services.

The *Medicare Claims Processing Manual* states that NPPs may provide and be paid for CPO as long as the NPP had a collaborative arrangement with the physician who signed the initial certification. The requirements below apply to the NPP who is billing for CPO, as long as that collaborative arrangement exists. Here are other provider requirements to bill CPO.

- The physician may not have a significant financial arrangement with the Home Health Agency (HHA) or hospice that is providing care to the patient;
- The physician may not be an employee or medical director of the HHA or hospice, even on a voluntary basis;
- Only one physician per month may bill and be paid for CPO and it must be the physician who signed the certification for home health or hospice;
- The physician must have had a face-to-face E/M service with the patient in the past six months; and
- The physician must personally provide 30 minutes of service in a calendar month.

For an NPP to bill CPO for a patient receiving home health services:
- The physician and NPP must be in the same group; or
- If the NPP is a Nurse Practitioner or Clinical Nurse Specialist, the physician signing the plan of care has a collaborative relationship with the NPP; or

- If the NPP is a physician assistant, the physician signing the plan of care is also the physician who provides general supervision of the PA;
- The NPP must have seen and examined the patient;
- The NPP providing the CPO is not a consultant caring for a single medical condition; and
- The NPP providing CPO integrates his or her care with the physician's care.

For hospice CPO, the attending physician or nurse practitioner may only bill if she is designated by the patient as the attending physician when the patient signs up for hospice. She may not be employed by the hospice provider.

Beneficiary Requirements

To receive CPO services, the beneficiary or patient must also meet certain criteria. The beneficiary:

- Must be receiving Medicare-covered HHA or hospice services during the period in which CPO is billed; and
- The beneficiary must require complex or multidisciplinary care modalities that necessitate ongoing physician involvement in the patient's treatment and plan of care.

Clinical Examples

A patient with poorly controlled diabetes develops a non-healing skin ulcer of the foot. The physician sees the patient in the office for this complaint and certifies the patient for services in a Medicare-enrolled Home Health Agency. The physician also arranges for services at a Wound Care Center and discusses the patient's care with the treating physician at the Wound Care Center. Over the next month, the physician reviews multiple lab results (not connected to an office visit), adjusts the patient's medications, and has multiple phone conversations with the nursing staff of the HHA and the physician at the Wound Care Center. The physician documents the date, time spent, and description of the work in a log kept in the patient's medical record. The physician signs the log. At the end of the month, the time spent is 45 minutes, which is over the threshold time of 30 minutes or more. The physician bills Medicare one unit using G0181, and using the first and last dates of the calendar month as the start date and the end date for the service. The staff indicates the provider number of the HHA on the claim form.

A Nurse Practitioner (NP) provides ongoing medical care to a patient who is being treated for colon cancer. This NP is employed by an Internal Medicine group. The patient is receiving chemotherapy at a tertiary care facility 30 miles away. The NP sees the patient regularly for other chronic medical problems. At a regularly scheduled follow-up visit, the patient complains of fatigue, loss of appetite, and pain. The NP decides that home health services are needed to manage the patient, and her collaborating physician completes the certifying plan of care for the HHA. During the course of the next month, the NP arranges for nutrition services, talks to the nursing staff at the HHA, discusses the patient's care with the Oncologist treating the patient, reviews lab work not related to an E/M visit, and makes adjustments to the patient's care. At the end of the month, the time spent in all of these activities is 60 minutes, over the required 30 minutes of time needed to bill CPO. Although the NP had extensive conversations with the patient's daughter over the phone during the course of the month, the time spent in discussion with the patient's family is not included on the log or included in the time used to meet the threshold time to bill CPO. These discussions are documented in the patient record but excluded from the calculation of time for CPO. The NP bills Medicare one unit of CPO, G0181, using the first and last days of the month as the start and end date for the service. The staff indicates the provider number of the HHA on the claim form.

Service Components

Care plan oversight is a time-based code. All time-based codes require that the time spent be documented in the patient's clinical record, not just in the billing record. Other examples of time-based codes include critical care, prolonged services, discharge visit 99239, and E/M services when time is the determining factor in selecting the code. Like critical care, specific activities may and may not be counted in the time billed for the service. You can count these provider activities in the time spent in CPO:

- Development of or revision of care plans;
- Review of subsequent reports;
- Review of diagnostic studies if the review is not part of an E/M service;
- Telephone calls with other health care professionals who are not employees of the practice and who are involved in the patient's care;
- Team conferences;

- Discussions with a pharmacist about drug treatment and interactions (not routine prescription renewals);
- Activities to coordinate care if physician or NPP time is required; and
- Making and implementing changes to the treatment plan.

Services Not Countable as CPO

There also are specific activities that may seem like CPO to the provider, but which may not be included in the time in determining whether the threshold 30 minutes was met in any single month. Be sure that the log or documentation that you use is specific enough to allow the staff to determine whether the activities are countable or not.

You may not count these activities in the time used to bill CPO:
- Time spent in routine renewing of prescriptions, whether performed by staff or provider;
- Time spent talking with an employee of the practice;
- Time spent by non-provider (MD or NPP) employees of the practice in CPO activities;
- Travel time by anyone;
- Time spent preparing or submitting claims or calculating the CPO time;
- Time spent talking to the patient's family, even if discussing treatment plan changes;
- Informal consults with physicians who are not treating the patient;
- Work of discharge visits, 99217, 99238, 99239;
- Interpretation of test results at E/M visit; or
- Routine post-operative care in the global period.

Billing Rules

Bill CPO on a monthly basis using the first and last date of the calendar month as the dates of service. Bill for one unit, no matter how much time you spent doing CPO for that patient. Make sure you have documented that you reached the threshold time of 30 minutes for the service that month. You must include the provider number of the HHA or hospice on your claim form.

Your physician, or the physician with whom the NPP has a collaborative arrangement, must have certified the patient for home health or hospice services in order to be paid.

Keeping Track

Some practices have developed a patient log that they keep in the chart. This allows the physician or NPP to document each instance in the month that they perform a CPO service. Include as headings on the log, the date the service was provided, the service, and the time spent on that date. The provider must sign the log. The practice must also keep a separate listing of patients on whom the provider is doing CPO services so they can look in the chart at the end of the month and see if the total time is over 30 minutes.

WHY DOES THE OIG CARE?

Here is the entry from the Office of Inspector General Work Plan for 2006 about care plan oversight:

> We will evaluate the efficacy of controls over Medicare payments for care plan oversight claims submitted by physicians. Care plan oversight exists where there is physician supervision of patients in hospice care that require complex or multidisciplinary modalities involving regular physician and/or revision of care plans. Reimbursement for care plan oversight increased from $15 million in 2000 to $41 million in 2001. We will assess whether these services were provided in accordance with Medicare regulations.
>
> *(OAS; W-00-04-35114; various reviews; expected issue date: FY 2006; work in progress)*

CMS saw a large increase in the payments for care plan oversight codes in a single year. Many physicians learned about the codes and began billing for them. However, the regulations are complex and the OIG wants to be sure that these services are being billed "in accordance with Medicare regulations."

If you provide and bill for CPO, it is worth the time to review the regulations and to audit for compliance with these regulations. The components of the service are complex and can be a confusing to both physicians and billers.

RED FLAGS

If you are billing for CPO, be sure your providers and staff understand the complex billing rules. Your biggest risk for this service is billing without knowing the rules. Take the time to ask a few providers these questions. If they don't know the answers, that is a warning to you.

- Can you include time spent talking to family members in your CPO services? (No)
- Do you have to sign your CPO log? (Yes)
- Are you keeping a written record of the date, time spent, and activity? (You must do this.)
- Can you include time spent talking to the pharmacist in your CPO service time? (Not for routine prescription renewals, but yes for discussion of benefits, risks, side effects of medicines.)
- Can you include the time you spent interacting with your own staff, hearing about phone messages, and asking your staff to perform services beneficial to this patient? (No. Time spent with your own staff may not be included, and their time in activities may not be included.)
- Do you count the time you spent calculating CPO time for billing in your CPO time? (No)
- Can you include the time spent in discharge services in CPO time? (No)

If your providers do not answer the above questions correctly, it is time for education and auditing. As the manager of the practice or billing department, make sure to look at the audit sheet and be sure the physician and beneficiary requirements are met. Those issues are covered on the audit sheet.

COMPLIANCE SOLUTIONS

If you do not have a log sheet to help your providers document the provision of CPO, develop one. Review the requirements listed in this chapter as you develop the audit sheet. Some practices print it on two-part NCR paper. One copy stays in the patient chart and one copy goes to the billing department at the end of the month. If you are using an EMR, a template can help a clinician keep track of this.

Develop a procedure to track patients who are eligible for CPO. The physician will need to generate the list for you to start or you might be able to track patients who are under the care of a Home Health Agency or hospice. Of course, not all patients under the care of home health or hospice are eligible for CPO, but to receive CPO, the patient must be under the care of one of those programs. Then, the physician or NPP can add names to the list of patients who might receive CPO. The physician or NPP will need to let the billing department know that he is providing CPO services to an eligible patient. At the end of the month, someone from billing will collect the second part of the NCR log and see if the total time for the month was 30 minutes. If so, bill for the service. If not, you can discard the billing copy of the log. The original remains in the patient chart documenting the work done by the physician or NPP.

COMPLIANCE PLAN AUDIT SHEET

Auditor Name:	Date of Audit:
Organization Name:	

Care Plan Oversight

To perform this audit, you will need:
- The medical record for each visit
- Access to the patient account
- Knowledge of employment and collaborative agreements

Select 10 patients for whom G0181 or G0182 were billed

Patient ID:		Physician ID:	
Date of Service:	Auditor ID:		Date of Audit:

You must answer YES to questions 1–6 to bill G0181 or G0182.

1. Is the patient receiving Medicare-covered home health services or is the patient enrolled in a Medicare-covered hospice program?	☐ Yes	⭕ No
2. Is the patient condition complex, or does it require multiple medical modalities?	☐ Yes	⭕ No
3. Was the patient seen by the provider for an E/M service in the past six months?	☐ Yes	⭕ No
4. If provided by an NPP, is there a collaborative agreement with the physician or are they in the same practice?	☐ Yes	⭕ No
5. If the physician provided the CPO, was it the same physician who signed the original plan of care?	☐ Yes	⭕ No
6. Is more than 30 minutes in a calendar month documented in a signed log, with a description of the activity?	☐ Yes	⭕ No

Do not bill if you answer YES to any question between numbers 7 and 10.

7. Does the physician have a financial relationship with the HHA?	☐ Yes	⭕ No
8. Is the physician the medical director or an employee of the hospice?	☐ Yes	⭕ No
9. Did the physician bill ESRD capitation for this patient, this month?	☐ Yes	⭕ No
10. If the patient is in a global surgical period, is this service related to the surgery?	☐ Yes	⭕ No

The CPO service must be documented in the record. You must answer YES to these questions, based on the documentation:		
11. Does the service document review of charts, reports, treatment plans, lab studies, medical decision making, physician activities to coordinate services, telephone calls with other health care professionals, team conferences?	☐ Yes	○ No
12. Does the medical record show the dates and times the service was provided?	☐ Yes	○ No
13. Is the time 30 minutes or more total for the month?	☐ Yes	○ No
14. Did you bill with the start and end date of the month?	☐ Yes	○ No
15. Are the specific activities performed documented?	☐ Yes	○ No
16. Is the record signed by the provider?	☐ Yes	○ No

CHAPTER 14

Transitional Care Management (TCM) and Chronic Care Management (CCM)

Transitional Care Management

In 2013, Centers for Medicare and Medicaid Services (CMS) began paying for Transitional Care Management (TCM) services. These are services provided to patients who are transitioning from a facility to a non-facility. The services include one evaluation and management service and non–face-to-face services for 29 days after discharge. The patient must be discharged from inpatient care, observation status, a nursing facility or partial hospitalization to home, independent assisted living, or domiciliary care. Not all patients are eligible. These services are for new or established patients with moderate or high complexity medical decision making who have medical or psychosocial problems that require extra care to manage the transition from the facility to home.

The service requires that someone from the physician office call the patient within two business days of discharge. The billing clinician, who can be a physician or a non-physician practitioner must review the discharge summary. The patient is seen in the office in seven or fourteen calendar days. Medication reconciliation and management must occur no later than the date of the face-to-face evaluation and management service. TCM then includes the work of clinical staff providing non–face-to-face care for the subsequent 29 days after discharge. The service is billed with the date of service that is 30 days from discharge, counting the day of discharge as day one.

According to CPT, these non–face-to-face services by the clinical staff during the 29-day post-discharge period include the following:
- Communication with the patient, caregiver, family, home health agency and/or other community services involved in the patient's care
- Education to support activities of daily living; assessment and support of the treatment regimen and medication management
- Identification of community and health resources and facilitating access to these resources

In addition to reviewing the discharge summary, the clinician will follow up on diagnostic tests, interact with other healthcare professionals involved in the patient's care, provide education of patient, family, or caregiver, and establish or reestablish referrals and assist in scheduling medical care or community care.

The first face-to-face service is not reported separately. Additional face-to-face services during the TCM period may be reported separately. The difference between 99495 and 99496 is first the complexity of the patient. At some time during the TCM period from the date of discharge until 30 days later, the patient must be of either moderate or high complexity medical decision making. This is determined using the criteria in the Documentation Guidelines. As a quick and dirty means of determining which code to report, use this: If the follow-up visit would have been a 99214, report 99495, whether the patient was seen in seven or 14 calendar days. If the follow-up visit would have been in 99215, indicating that the patient had high medical decision-making complexity and the patient was seen within seven calendar days, report a 99496 code.

99495: TCM services with the following required elements:

- Communication (direct contact, telephone, electronic) with the patient and/or caregiver within two business days of discharge
- Medical decision making of at least moderate complexity during the service period
- Face-to-face visit, within 14 calendar days of discharge
- 99496: Transitional Care Management Services with the following required elements:
- Communication (direct contact, telephone, electronic) with the patient and/or caregiver within two business days of discharge
- Medical decision making of at least high complexity during the service period
- Face-to-face visit, within seven calendar days of discharge

Other codes and services are bundled with Transitional Care Management. The codes that may not be billed with the TCM codes are the following:

- Care Plan Oversight (99339, 99340, 99474-99380, G0181, G0182)
- Prolonged services without patient contact (99358, 99359)
- Anticoagulant management (99363, 99364)
- Medical team conferences (99366–99368)
- Education and training (98960–98962, 99441–99443)
- End-stage renal disease services (90951–90970)
- Online medical evaluation (98969, 99444)

Preparation of special reports (99080), analysis of data (99090, 99091), complex care coordination services (99487–99489), or medication therapy services (99605–99607) during the time period covered by the TCM codes, which is 29 days after discharge. Of course, Medicare does not reimburse many of the codes in the list above. The new chronic care management code 99490 is also bundled with Transitional Care Management.

KEY POINTS

Date of service	Count the discharge as day one; use DOS 30 on the claim form.
Place of service	Place where face-to-face service took place.
What about readmissions?	TCM may not be reported for overlapping periods. Select one of the admissions, and report TCM for the 30-day period starting the day of the discharge.
Who can perform the face-to-face E/M service?	Physician, NP, PA, or a Clinical Nurse Specialist can perform this, i.e., people who are qualified to perform an E/M service within their scope of practice.
Is it moderate or high complexity and when?	Any time during the TCM period
What if there additional office visits exist?	Report (bill for) other office visits after the first bundled TCM service.

Chronic Care Management (CCM)

The CMS is committed to providing increased support for primary care services. They recognize the significant work in managing the care of chronically ill patients that takes place between office visits on a day when there is no face-to-face service with the patient. CMS is using 99490, which is a new CPT code for chronic care management. Other chronic care management codes are in the CPT book, e.g., 99487 and 99489, have a status indicator of bundled, and Medicare does not pay for them.

99490: Chronic care management (CCM) services, at least 20 minutes of clinical staff time directed by a physician or other qualified health care professional, per calendar month, with the following required elements:

- Multiple (two or more) chronic conditions expected to last at least 12 months or until the death of the patient

- Chronic conditions place the patient at significant risk of death, acute exacerbation/decompensation, or functional decline
- Comprehensive care plan established, implemented, revised, or monitored

Scope of services:

- 24-hour-a-day, 7-day-a-week access to the practice (on-call)
- Continuity of care with a designated practitioner and able to get successive routine appointments with that provider
- Care management for chronic conditions including the following: systematic assessment of the patient's medical, functional, and psychosocial needs; system-based approaches to ensure timely receipt of all recommended preventive care services; medication reconciliation with review of adherence and potential interactions; and oversight of patient self-management of medications

In consultation with the patient, any caregiver and other key practitioners treating the patient, the provider must create a patient-centered care plan document to assure care is provided in a way that is congruent with patient choices and values. The care plan is based on a physical, mental, cognitive, psychosocial, functional, and environmental (re)assessment and an inventory of resources and supports. This comprehensive plan of care for all health issues typically includes, but is not limited to, the following elements:

- Problem list
- Expected outcome and prognosis
- Measurable treatment goals
- Symptom management
- Planned interventions
- Medication management
- Community/social services ordered
- How the services of agencies and specialists unconnected to the billing practice will be directed/coordinated
- Identification of the individuals responsible for each intervention
- Requirements for periodic review and, when applicable, revision of the care plan

A full list of problems, medications, and medication allergies in the electronic health record (EHR) must inform the care plan, care coordination, and ongoing clinical care. The service includes management of care transition, electronic exchange of information, and a goal of reducing readmissions.

- Coordination with home-based and community-based clinical service. Communication to and from home-based and community-based providers regarding these patient needs must be documented in the patient's medical record.
- Enhanced opportunities for the beneficiary and any relevant caregiver to communicate with the practitioner regarding the beneficiary's care through telephone access and the use of secure messaging, the Internet, or other asynchronous non–face-to-face consultation methods.

Additional Medicare requirements:

- Inform the beneficiary about the availability of the CCM services from the practitioner and obtains his or her written agreement to have the services provided, including the beneficiary's authorization for the electronic communication of the patient's medical information with other treating providers as part of care coordination.
- Document in the beneficiary's medical record that all elements of the CCM service were explained and offered to the beneficiary, and note the beneficiary's decision to accept or decline the service.
- Provide the beneficiary a written or electronic copy of the care plan and document in the electronic medical record that the care plan was provided to the beneficiary.
- Inform the beneficiary of the right to stop the CCM services at any time (effective at the end of a calendar month) and the effect of a revocation of the agreement to receive CCM services.
- Inform the beneficiary that only one practitioner can furnish and be paid for these services during the calendar month service period.

According to CPT, a practice may not count clinical staff time performed on the same day as these E/M services (99201–99215, 99324–99328, 99334–99397, 99341–99350) Office visits, rest home services, home services.

Bundled services with CCM

CCM 99490 may not be reported during the month the practice reports the following:

- Care Plan Oversight 99339, 99340, 99374—99380, G0181, G0182

- Non–face-to-face prolonged care 99358, 99359
- Anticoagulant management 99363, 99364
- Medical team conferences 99366, 99367, 99368,
- Education and training 98960, 98961, 98962, 99071, 99078
- Telephone services 99366, 99367, 99368, 99441, 99442, 99443
- Online medical evaluation 98969, 99444
- Preparation of special reports 99080
- Analysis of data 99090, 99091
- Transitional care management services 99495, 99496
- Medication therapy management services 99605, 99606, 99607

Do not report 99490 if reporting end-stage renal dialysis services 90951–90970 during the same month.

The surgeon may not report CCM during the postoperation period, during which the surgery has been performed.

Clinical staff

The non–face-to-face time that comprises the 20 minutes of CCM must be performed by clinical staff (per CPT and CMS). Though neither CPT nor CMS have defined clinical staff for us, it certainly includes registered nurses, licensed practical nurses (LPNs), and clinical care managers. In most states, medical assistants are licensed or certified. *Receptionists, schedulers and front desk staff are not clinical staff.* The time that nonclinical staff members spend making appointments or doing any follow-up would not be included in the clinical care management time.

Incident to

CMS has changed the rules for CCM and TCM related to incident to. The incident to the rules themselves have not changed, only the application to these two services has changed. The physician or non-physician practitioner who is billing CCM or TCM does not need to be in the suite of offices when the clinical staff is performing CCM-related services.

Patient informed consent form

The patient must give informed consent in writing prior to the start of reporting CCM services. The patient must be informed about the scope of the services and that he or she has the right to cancel them in any time. If the patient elects to cancel, the services would end at the end of that calendar month. This consent should also tell the patient that their electronic care plan will be shared with other health care professionals providing care during the period. The patient will be charged a co-pay and deductible for the service.

Electronic Health Record (EHR)

In consultation with the patient and the family member, a care plan must be established. This must be given to the patient electronically or in writing.

All practitioners and staff members whose minutes are counted for CCM must have electronic access to care plan.

Other team members must access the plan through secure messaging or a health exchange portal or through access to the electronic health record. Faxes are considered insufficient.

The practice must use certified EHR technology. For CCM payments in CY 2015, this policy will allow practitioners to use EHR technology certified to the 2011 or 2014 edition(s) of certification criteria.

Why does the Office of Inspector General (OIG) Care?

New services tend to have a high error rate particularly during the first two years. These services are complex, and the requirements are specific. Not all patients who are discharged from the hospital will be eligible for TCM services. Similarly, CCM is not a per-member, per-month benefit and may only be billed with the clinical staff time in the calendar month of 20 minutes or more.

The payment for TCM is also relatively high. This includes substantial practice expense relative value units (RVUs) because the clinical staff does much of the work. Some practices do not have a nurse in the office. Current procedural terminology (CPT) states a licensed clinical staff should do this work. The Centers for Medicare and Medicaid Services (CMS) noted this in its frequently asked questions document: "Medicare encourages practitioners to follow CPT guidance in reporting TCM services. Medicare requires that when a practitioner bills Medicare for services and supplies commonly furnished in physician offices, the practitioner must meet the 'incident to' requirements described in Chapter 15 (Section 60) of the Benefit Policy Manual 100-02." This section does not mandate require staff members who provide incident to services be licensed nurses. A group is more likely to be successful at these services if it has nurses in the office. Although the CCM payment is more modest, many primary care practices will have a large population of patients with two or more chronic illnesses. There is a potential for significant revenue if the practice is able to do the case management, comply with the EHR rules, and document 20 minutes of care per month.

RED FLAGS

Neither TMC nor CCM are on the OIG's Work Plan yet. I would consider it a red flag if all patients discharged were billed for Transitional Care Management. There are significant requirements that may be difficult to achieve every time. First, not all patients are medically and socially complicated. There could be some injuries or illnesses that require admission for which the patient does not require help in the transition between the facility and home. Second, practices may be unable to reach all patients by phone in two business days. Without that initial contact, the group may not bill for Transitional Care Management. A medical practice may not get notice in two days when patients are discharged from a tertiary care center. Also, the extra work and effort a practice thought would be needed to keep a patient out of the hospital may not be needed and is, therefore, not performed. If these non–face-to-face supportive services are not done and documented, do not bill for Transitional Care Management.

I would consider it a red flag if all patients signed up for CCM were billed in every month. Keep in mind that this is not a per-member, per-month benefit and may only be reported in a calendar month in which the clinical staff spends 20 minutes in the service.

COMPLIANCE RESPONSE

Review the rules for TCM and CCM with all providers, clinical staff and billing staff. Make sure a process is in place to call patients after they are discharged within two business days and to document the call. Document the review of the discharge summary, the medication reconciliation, and the extra non–face-to-face work performed after the office visit. (The first E/M service is typically in the office but could be in the home or an assisted living facility.)

For CCM, do not start reporting the service unless the practice has nursing and case management services in place. There needs to be the infrastructure to support the service. Many EHRs do not have the capability of a dynamic care plan, the means to document minutes of staff time, or the ability to allow non-practice team members access to the care plan electronically. Start by working on the structure and team needed to perform the services.

TRANSITIONAL CARE MANAGEMENT AUDIT SHEET

Patient ID:		Provider ID:		
Auditor ID:	Date of Audit:		DOS:	
For every service billed with 99495 or 99496 you must answer yes to these questions.				
1. Does the patient require coordination of care, education, or additional support in making the transition from the facility to home, and was the patient discharged from inpatient care, observation status, nursing facility or partial hospitalization?			☐ Yes	○ No
2. Is there documentation of a completed phone call within two business days?			☐ Yes	○ No
3. Is there documentation that the discharge summary was reviewed?			☐ Yes	○ No
4. Is there documentation that the medications were reconciled, no later than the E/M visit?			☐ Yes	○ No
5. Was an E/M service done in 7 calendar days for 99496 or 14 calendar days for 99495?			☐ Yes	○ No
6. Was the medical complexity high for 99496 or moderate for 99495?			☐ Yes	○ No
7. Is there evidence that staff provided non-face-to-face support such as communication (with patient, family members, guardian or caretaker, surrogate decision makers, and/or other professionals) regarding aspects of care, communication with home health agencies and other community services utilized by the patient, patient and/or family/caretaker education to support self-management, independent living, and activities of daily living, assessment and support for treatment regimen adherence and medication management, identification of available community and health resources, facilitating access to care and services needed by the patient and/or family?			☐ Yes	○ No
8. Is there documentation the provider performed non-face-to-face services such as obtaining and reviewing the discharge information (eg, discharge summary, as available, or continuity of care documents); reviewing need for or follow-up on pending diagnostic tests and treatments; interaction with other qualified health care professionals who will assume or reassume care of the patient's system-specific problems; education of patient, family, guardian, and/or caregiver; establishment or reestablishment of referrals and arranging for needed community resources; assistance in scheduling any required follow-up with community providers and services?			☐ Yes	○ No

CHRONIC CARE MANAGEMENT AUDIT SHEET

Patient ID:		Provider ID:	
Auditor ID:	Date of Audit:	DOS:	

For services reported with code 99490.

1. Does the patient have two or more chronic conditions expected to last at least 12 months or until the death of the patient which place the patient at significant risk of death, acute exacerbation/decompensation or functional decline?	❒ Yes	○ No
2. Is the practice using certified EHR technology?	❒ Yes	○ No
3. Do all team members have access to the care plan through the EHR, an HIE, web platform or secure messaging?	❒ Yes	○ No
4. Is informed consent documented in the medical record?	❒ Yes	○ No
5. Is a dynamic care plan documented in the chart? According to CPT: *A care plan is based on a physical, mental, cognitive, social, functional, and environmental assessment. It is a comprehensive plan of care for all health problems. It typically includes, but is not limited to, the following elements: problem list, expected outcome and prognosis, measurable treatment goals, symptom management, planned interventions, medication management, community/social services ordered, how the services of agencies and specialists unconnected to the practice will be directed/coordinated, identification of the individuals responsible for each intervention, requirements for periodic review, and, when applicable, revision of the care plan.*	❒ Yes	○ No
6. Are 20 minutes of non-face-to-face time by the clinical staff documented during the calendar month? According to CPT, these activities may include: *communication and engagement with patient, family members, guardian or caretaker, surrogate decision makers, and/or other professionals regarding aspects of care; communication with home health agencies and other community services utilized by the patient; collection of health outcomes data and registry documentation; patient and/or family/caregiver education to support self-management, independent living, and activities of daily living; assessment and support for treatment regimen adherence and medication management; identification of available community and health resources; facilitating access to care and services needed by the patient and/or family; management of care transitions not reported as part of transitional care management (99495, 99496); ongoing review of patient status, including review of laboratory and other studies not reported as part of an E/M service, noted above; development, communication, and maintenance of a comprehensive care plan.*	❒ Yes	○ No

Final Thoughts

Medical practices are groaning under the strain of meaningful use and reporting on quality measures through the Physician Quality Reporting System in a difficult reimbursement environment. Why should a practice devote time and resources to compliance? Watch the headlines in any national newspaper for the answer to that question. Every week, there are important stories on the front page and in the business section detailing healthcare fraud accusations or convictions and federal and state government commitment to protecting healthcare programs. The government and third-party payers are serious about finding and preventing fraud and abuse in healthcare claims. Both have a mandate to protect the finances of their funders: taxpayers and purchasers of healthcare. Medical practice leaders have an imperative duty to protect their practices with an effective compliance plan.

The Accountable Care Act included a provision that practices must return monies collected in error to the government within 60 days of discovering an overpayment. This adds urgency to medical practices' compliance activity. In September 2012 the Centers for Medicare & Medicaid Services (CMS) approved the first Recovery Audit Contractor to review E/M code 99215, the highest-level established patient visit. That same week, *The New York Times* reported that an analysis of Emergency Department (ED) billing showed that using electronic health records increased the level of service for ED services billed to Medicare. This in the wake of the May 2012 Office of Inspector General (OIG) report that showed the drift of Evaluation and Management codes from lower to higher during the past decade.

But, it is not just government payers who are reviewing the coding patterns of physician practices and auditing records. Many private payers are analyzing data and sending letters to physicians noting that their use of certain codes is higher than the norm or that their use of the certain modifier is too high. After that, it is very common for the payer to request records. All practices need to protect themselves.

Most large groups have a formal compliance plan and have designated a compliance officer. Annual reviews are part of their routine.

Some smaller practices may have ignored this obligation, thinking that having no compliance plan was safer than a compliance plan not followed. Those days are gone. There is no protection in not having a plan in place. If you do not have a plan, develop one and implement it. If you do have a plan, review it. Be sure that coders and providers attend coding education, that you perform internal or external annual audits, and that there is a process in place for investigating complaints or concerns.

Coding compliance, the subject of this book, is only one aspect of compliance. Be sure your privacy policies and procedures are up-to-date. Whoever does your hiring and manages human resources should check personnel files for signed code of conduct forms for all employees. A healthcare attorney should review all contracts, including employment, rent or lease agreements, and any other signed contract the practice has.

In one year, a group can't audit all of the areas covered in this book, and this book describes a small fraction of the areas of risk. Your practice may have another risk area that is critical to review such as diagnostic testing or use of Advance Beneficiary Notices. Select your risk areas by considering these factors:

- High volume services by dollar value, RVU, or volume;
- Unusual coding pattern when compared to CMS norms;
- A billing pattern that shows over 90% of all E/M charges in the highest two categories of E/M services;
- Newly adopted electronic health records (identical notes an issue);
- Non-physician practitioner billing; and
- Items on the OIG Work Plan that you perform.

It is not possible to look at all of those areas in a single year's audit. It is also not required that you look at the same items for each clinician. You may focus on different areas for different departments or different providers in a group. Don't steer away from an item that you know may be problematic out of fear of finding errors. It is better for the practice to find errors, correct them, educate and refund, rather than waiting for one of the many government watchdog organizations to find the errors.

Document your compliance policies and activities. If staff members attend educational sessions or listen to coding webinars, keep copies of the certificates in your compliance files. When reviewing your compliance plan, note everything you said you would do: have employees sign a code of conduct; perform audits; provide education. When you complete those activities in a year, document that you have done so.

Medical practices feel squeezed by expenses without much in the way of increases in fee allowances. Now is not the time to cut costs in coding, billing, and compliance education for anyone. That $2,000 spent to send a key staff member or physician leader to a coding seminar could produce revenue or save you thousands of dollars in payback and fines. Webinars that everyone can attend for a single fee are an economical way to use education dollars.

Specialty societies are a terrific source of up-to-date information about coding and billing. Physicians who are members of their societies can often get three to five free coding questions answered. The societies send e-mail updates. Use these resources.

And finally, when you have performed an audit, follow up on the results. The single biggest mistake I see is not following up on audit results. A group hires an external auditor who identifies an error. Not a "stop the presses, go directly to jail error" but an error that requires a refund and education. Do the refund and educate staff and clinicians. Then, a month later, look again. Has the problem stayed solved and corrected?

A physician has an obligation to "first, do no harm." Medical practice leaders have an obligation to protect their practices from harm by actively instituting an effective compliance plan. This book provides one resource for practices: accurate coding information and compliance sheets for high-risk coding.

Your Nicoletti Auditing Physician Services Audit Worksheets are available at:

http://auditing2.greenbranch.com

Code: J6G37E

Download Audit Worksheets at http://auditing2.greenbranch.com
Access code printed on page 195 of this book

E/M Documentation Auditing Worksheet

Provider Name:

Patient ID:

Date of Service:

CPT Codes Billed:

CPT Codes Audited:

ICD-9 Codes Billed:

ICD-9 Codes Audited:

Path Note?

Path Error?

Other Issues:

Auditor Name:

E/M Documentation Auditing Worksheet

Provider Name:

Patient ID:

Date of Service:

CPT Codes Billed:

CPT Codes Audited:

ICD-9 Codes Billed:

ICD-9 Codes Audited:

Path Note?

Path Error?

Other Issues:

Auditor Name:

Chief Complaint:

H I S T O R Y	**HPI (history of present illness)** ❑ Location ❑ Severity ❑ Timing ❑ Modifying factors ❑ Quality ❑ Duration ❑ Context ❑ Associated signs and symptoms				Brief	Brief 1-3 elements	Extended	Extended ≥ 4 elements or status of 3 chronic or inactive conditions
	ROS (review of systems) ❑ Constitutional ❑ Ears, Nose, ❑ GI ❑ Integumentary ❑ Endo (wt loss, etc) Mouth, Throat ❑ GU (skin, breast) ❑ Hem/lymph ❑ Eyes ❑ Card/vasc ❑ Musculo ❑ Neuro ❑ All/imm ❑ Resp ❑ Psych ❑ "All others negative"				None	Pertinent to problem 2-9 systems 1 system	Extended 2-9 systems	Complete ≥ 10 systems, or some systems with statement "all others negative"
	PFSH (past, family, and social history) ❑ Past Medical History ❑ Family History			Established/ER	None	None	One history area	Two or three history areas
	❑ Social History No PFSH required: 99231-33, 99307-99310			New/ Consult/ Admit	None	None	One or two history area(s)	Three history areas
	Circle the entry farthest to the right for each history area. To determine history level, draw a line down the column with the circle farthest to the left.				**PROBLEM FOCUSED**	**EXP. PROB. FOCUSED**	**DETAILED**	**COMPRE-HENSIVE**

1995 and 1997 Multi-specialty Exams on next page.

Remember: if you use the status of three chronic diseases for the HPI, you must use one of the 1997 exams: either the multi-specialty exam or one of the single system exams.

A | Number of Diagnoses or Treatment Options

Problems to Exam Physician	Number X	Points	= Result
Self-limited or minor (stable, improved or worsening)		1	Max=2
Est. problem (to examiner); stable, improved		1	
Est. problem (to examiner); worsening		2	
New problem (to examiner); no additional workup planned		3	Max=3
New prob. (to examiner); add. workup planned		4	
		TOTAL	

Bring total to **line A** in Final Result for Complexity

B | Amount and/or Complexity of Data to Be Reviewed

Data to Be Reviewed	Points
Review and/or order of clinical lab tests	1
Review and/or order of tests in the radiology section of the CPT	1
Review and/or order of tests in the medicine section of the CPT	1
Discussion of test results with performing physician	1
Decision to obtain old records and/or obtain history from someone other than patient	1
Review and summarization of old records and/or obtaining history from someone other than patient and/or discussion of case with another health care provider	2
Independent visualization of image, tracing or specimen itself (not simply review of report)	2
	TOTAL

Bring total to **line B** in Final Result for Complexity

Final Result of Complexity

Draw a line down the column with 2 or 3 circles and circle decision making level OR draw a line down the column with the center circle and circle the decision-making level.

A	Number of diagnoses or treatment options	≤ 1 minimal	2 Limited	3 Multiple	≥ 4 Extensive
B	Amount and complexity of data	≤ 1 minimal or low	2 Limited	3 Moderate	≥ 4 Extensive
C	Highest risk	Minimal	Low	Moderate	High
	Type or decision making	STRAIGHT FORWARD	LOW COMPLEX	MODERATE COMPLEX	HIGH COMPLEX

C | Risk of Complications and/or Morbidity or Mortality

LEVEL OF RISK	Presenting Problem(s)	Diagnostic Procedure(s) Ordered	Management Options Selected
MINIMAL	• One self-limited or minor problem, e.g. cold, insect bite, tinea corporis	• Laboratory tests requiring venipuncture • Chest x-rays • EKG/EEG • Urinalysis • Ultrasound, e.g. echo • KOH prep	• Rest • Gargles • Elastic bandages • Superficial dressings
LOW	• Two or more self-limited or minor problems • One stable chronic illness, e.g. well controlled hypertension, non-insulin dependent diabetes, cataract, BPH • Acute uncomplicated illness or injury, e.g. cystitis, allergic rhinitis, simple sprain	• Physiologic tests not under stress, e.g. pulm. function tests • Non-cardiovascular imaging studies with contrast, e.g. barium enema • Superficial needle biopsies • Clinical laboratory tests requiring arterial puncture • Skin biopsies	• Over-the-counter drugs • Minor surgery with no identified risk factors • Physical therapy • IV fluids without additives
MODERATE	• One or more chronic illnesses with mild exacerbation, progression, or side effects of treatment • Two or more stable chronic illnesses • Undiagnosed new problem with uncertain prognosis, e.g. lump in breast • Acute illness with systemic symptoms, e.g. pyelonephritis, pneumonitis, colitis • Acute complicated injury, e.g. head injury with brief loss of consciousness	• Physiologic tests under stress, e.g. cardiac stress test, fetal contraction stress test • Diagnostic endoscopies with no identified risk factors • Deep needle or incisional biopsy • Cardiovascular imaging studies with contrast and no identified risk factors, e.g. arteriogram, cardiac cath • Obtain fluid from body cavity, e.g. lumbar puncture, thoracentesis, culdocentesis	• Minor surgery with identified risk factors • Elective major surgery (open, percutaneous or endoscopic) with no identified risk factors • Prescription drug management • Therapeutic nuclear medicine • IV fluids with additives • Closed treatment of fracture or dislocation without manipulation
HIGH	• One or more chronic illnesses with severe exacerbation, progression, or side effects of tx • Acute or chronic illnesses or injuries that may pose a threat to life or bodily function, e.g. multiple trauma, acute MI, pulmonary embolus, severe respiratory distress, progressive severe rheumatoid arthritis, psychiatric illness with potential threat to self or others, peritonitis, acute renal failure • An abrupt change in neurologic status, e.g. seizure, TIA, weakness or sensory loss	• Cardiovascular imaging studies with contrast with identified risk factors • Cardiac electrophysiological tests • Diagnostic endoscopies with identified risk factors • Discography	• Elective major surgery (open, percutaneous or endoscopic) with identified risk factors • Emergency major surgery (open, percutaneous or endoscopic) • Parenteral controlled substances • Drug therapy requiring intensive monitoring for toxicity • Decision not to resuscitate or to de-escalate care because of poor prognosis

Bring total to **line C** in Final Result for Complexity

1995 Multi-specialty Exam

1995	Organ systems:					Body area or system related to problem	2-7 systems Limited	2-7 systems Extended	8 or more systems not body parts
	❏ Constitutional (e.g. vitals, gen app) ❏ Eyes	❏ Ears, Nose, Mouth, Throat ❏ Cardiovascular	❏ Resp ❏ GI ❏ GU	❏ Musclo ❏ Skin ❏ Neuro	❏ Psych ❏ Hem/lymph/Imm ❏ Affected body area				
						PROBLEM FOCUSED	EXP. PROB. FOCUSED	DETAILED	COMPRE-HENSIVE

Body Areas

1) Head, including the face
2) Neck
3) Chest, including breasts and axillae
4) Abdomen
5) Genitalia, groin and buttocks
6) Back, including spine
7) Each extremity

Problem focused: 1995 guidelines: a limited examination of the affected body area or organ system (1 element)

Expanded problem focused: 1995 guidelines: a limited examination of the affected body area or organ system and other symptomatic or related organ systems (2-7 elements)

Detailed: 1995 guidelines: an extended examination of the affected body area(s) and other symptomatic or related organ system(s) (2-7 elements)

Comprehensive: 1995 guidelines: a general multi-system exam or complete examination of a single organ system (8 elements)

1997 Multi-specialty Exam

		Problem Focused AT LEAST 1 from any systems/areas	Exp Problem Focused AT LEAST 6 from any systems/areas	Detailed AT LEAST 12 from at least 2 systems/areas	Comprehensive AT LEAST 18 from at least 9 systems/areas
E X A M I N A T I O N	Constitutional:	❏ Any three vital signs	❏ General appearance of patient		
	Eyes:	❏ Conjunctivae & lids	❏ Pupils & irises	❏ Optic discs	
	ENT:	❏ External ears & nose ❏ Oropharynx	❏ EACs & TMs	❏ Hearing ❏ Nasal mucosa, septum & turbinates	❏ Lips, teeth & gums
	Neck:	❏ Neck ❏ Thyroid			
	Resp:	❏ Respiratory effort	❏ Percussion	❏ Palpation	❏ Auscultation
	CV:	❏ Palpation of heart ❏ Pedal pulses	❏ Auscultation ❏ Extremities for edema &/or varicosities	❏ Carotids	❏ Abdominal aorta ❏ Femoral
	Chest (Breasts):	❏ Inspection of breasts	❏ Palpation of breasts & axillae		
	GI (Abdomen):	❏ Masses, tenderness	❏ Liver & spleen	❏ Hernia	❏ Anus, perineum & rectum ❏ Occult test
	GU:	Male: ❏ Scrotal contents Female: ❏ External genitalia	❏ Penis ❏ Urethra	❏ Prostate gland ❏ Bladder	❏ Cervix ❏ Uterus ❏ Adnexa/parametria
	Lymph:	❏ Lymph nodes in two or more areas:		❏ Neck ❏ Axillae ❏ Groin ❏ Other	
	Musculoskeletal:	❏ Gait & Station	❏ Digits & Nails		

	H/N	Sp	LA	RA	LL	RL	Exam of joints, bones muscle in:
							Inspect &/or palpate-note any misalignment, tenderness, masses
							Range of motion (SLR, pain, etc.)
							Stability (subluxation, laxity, etc.)
							Muscle strength or tone

Skin	❏ Inspection of skin & subcutaneous tissue ❏ Palpation of skin & subcutaneous tissue
Neuro:	❏ Cranial nerves ❏ Reflexes ❏ Sensation
Psych:	❏ Judgment & Insight ❏ Orientation to time, place & person ❏ Memory ❏ Mood & affect

Transfer the history, exam and medical decision making results to the appropriate chart below and follow the specific instructions for that chart.

PF = Problem focused   *EPF* = Expanded Problem Focused   *D* = Detailed   *C* = Comprehensive
SF = Straightforward   *L* = Low   *M* = Moderate   *H* = High

LEVL OF SERVICE

Outpatient, Consultants (Outpatient, Inpatient & Confirmatory)

	New/Consults					Established				
	If a column has 3 circles, draw a line down the column and circle the code OR find the column with the circle farthest to the left, draw a line down the column and circle the code.					If a column has 2 or 3 circles, draw a line down the column and circle the code OR draw a line down the column with the center circle and circle the code.				
History	PF	EPF	D	C	C	Minimal	PF	EPF	D	C
Examination	PF	EPF	D	C	C	problem that may not require	PF	EPF	D	C
Complexity of medical decision	SF	SF	L	M	H	presence of physician	SF	L	M	H
	99201-10 99241-15 99251-20	99202-20 99242-30 99252-40	99203-30 99243-40 99253-55	99204-45 99244-60 99254-80	99205-60 99245-80 99255-110	99211 5	99212 10	99213 15	99214 25	99215 40

Inpatient

	Initial Hospital/Observation			Subsequent Inpatient		
	If a column has 3 circles, draw a line down the column and circle the code OR find the column with the circle farthest to the left, draw a line down the column and circle the code.			If a column has 2 or 3 circles, draw a line down the column and circle the code OR draw a line down the column with the center circle and circle the code.		
History	D or C	C	C	PF Interval	EPF Interval	D Interval
Examination	D or C	C	C	PF	EPF	D
Complexity of medical decision	SF/L	M	H	SF/L	M	H
	99221-30 99218-N/A 99234-N/A	99222-50 99219-N/A 99235-N/A	99223-70 99220-N/A 99236-N/A	99231-15	99232-25	99233-35

Nursing Facility

	Annual	Admission			Subsequent Nursing Facility			
		If a column has 3 circles, draw a line down the column and circle the code OR find the column with the circle farthest to the left, draw a line down the column and circle the code.			If a column has 2 or 3 circles, draw a line down the column and circle the code OR draw a line down the column with the center circle and circle the code.			
History	D Interval	D or C	C	C	PF Interval	EPF Interval	D Interval	C Interval
Examination	C	D or C	C	C	PF	EPF	D	C
Complexity of medical decision	L/M	SF/L	M	H	SF	L	M	H
	99318	99304	99305	99306	99307	99308	099309	99310

ER

	ER				
	If a column has 3 circles, draw a line down the column and circle the code OR find the column with the circle farthest to the left, draw a line down the column and circle the code.				
History	PF	EPF	EPF	D	C
Examination	PF	EPF	EPF	D	C
Complexity of medical decision	SF	L	M	M	H
	99281-N/A	99282-N/A	99283-N/A	99284-N/A	99285-N/A

TIME

If the physician documents total time and suggests that counseling or coordinating care dominates (more than 50%) the encounter, time may determine level of service. Documentation may refer to: prognosis, differential diagnosis, risks, benefits of treatment, instructions, compliance, risk reduction, or discussion with another health care provider.

Does documentation reveal total time? Time: Face-to-face in outpatient setting / Unit/Floor in inpatient setting	☐ Yes	☐ No	If all answers are "yes," may select level based on time.
Does documentation describe the content of counseling or coordinating care?	☐ Yes	☐ No	
Does documentation reveal that more than half of time was counseling or coordinating care?	☐ Yes	☐ No	

Index

audit sheet, 191
codes, billing avoidance, 184
compliance response, 190
details, 185
services, elements, 184
warning signs, 190
Treatment options, documentation example, 199

U

Unit time, importance, 58–59
Unremarkable (ROS), 40
Urgent Care Center, initiation, 65
U.S. Trust Fund, x

V

Visits
category/subcategory, relationship, 22
time, determining factor, 57–58

W

Walk-in clinic, initiation, 65
Word processing program, macros (usage problems), 56
Work Plan, 121
absence, 106
Wound Care Center services, 175